D1443480

face to face

face to face

My Quest to Perform the World's First Full Face Transplant

Maria Siemionow, MD, PhD

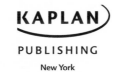

PUBLISHING

New York

Face to Face is based on real events; however, some names and other details have been changed to protect people's privacy.

Published by Kaplan Publishing, a division of Kaplan, Inc.
1 Liberty Plaza, 24th Floor
New York, NY 10006

Printed in the United States of America

Library of Congress Cataloging-in-Publication Data

Siemionow, Maria Z.
    Face to face : my quest to perform the world's first full face transplant / Maria Siemionow.
        p. ; cm.
    ISBN 978-1-60714-051-1 (alk. paper)
    1. Siemionow, Maria Z. 2. Face--Transplantation. 3. Surgeons--Biography. I. Title.
    [DNLM: 1. Siemionow, Maria Z. 2. Physicians--Poland--Personal Narratives.
3. Physicians--United States--Personal Narratives. 4. Facial Transplantation--
Poland. 5. Facial Transplantation--United States. 6. Surgery, Plastic--Poland--
Personal Narratives. 7. Surgery, Plastic--United States--Personal Narratives.
    WZ 100 S5723f 2009]
    RD523.S44 2009
    617.5'20592092--dc22
    [B]
                                                          2009001450

10 9 8 7 6 5 4 3 2 1

ISBN-13: 978-1-6071-0511

Kaplan Publishing books are available at special quantity discounts to use for sales promotions, employee premiums, or educational purposes. Please email our Special Sales Department to order or for more information at kaplanpublishing@kaplan.com, or write to Kaplan Publishing, 1 Liberty Plaza, 24th Floor, New York, NY 10006.

CONTENTS

INTRODUCTION

LOOK IN THE MIRROR. You see your face, sleepy in the morning, tired in the evening, capable of a thousand emotions — one or more for every experience, every encounter. Desire. Weariness. Irritation. Happiness. Sadness. Resignation. Joy. Even thoughts are reflected by a flicker here, a shift there. No other aspect of our anatomy is capable of even a fraction of the complexity of motion and emotion allowed by the muscles and tissues of the face.

The surface of the face has as many as 27 different landmarks on each side that give it character and help identify structures such as nerves and blood vessels that lie underneath. If you placed your fingertip in the middle of your upper lips and traced halfway around your mouth to the skin between your lower lip and chin, you would have crossed ten different muscles in that short trip. These muscles, which lie directly beneath the skin and control the movements of the mouth, cause everything from smiling to whistling to puckering up for a kiss to spitting out a watermelon seed. The eyes, the nose, the cheeks, and even the ears are controlled by a similar pattern of overlying muscles that pull the flesh in all directions. Thus the face can convey emotion, expression.

Imagine, however, if you looked in the mirror and saw something entirely different. Scars. Skin and tissue distorted by a burn. Lips reduced to a circle. And what if what was reflected back at you did not even register those emotions? What if your face was unable to move — it had been rendered a mask? What if you couldn't recognize yourself in the mirror? If that face — or what was left of it — stared back at you as if it were a stranger, how would you feel?

Most of us take for granted the value of our own face. We don't consciously realize how it reinforces and shapes our identity. When we look into a mirror, we assign an identity to the reflection, and that identity carries a great deal of weight. The reflection says this is a young person or an aging person, a successful person, a person with a goal, a person someone can love. Or perhaps this is someone whose visage is so scarred and distorted that even self-love seems impossible.

IN NOVEMBER 2004, Cleveland Clinic and I attracted worldwide attention when the hospital's institutional review board announced that it considered a face transplant to be both ethical and possible. The Clinic is used to such attention. I wasn't. Calls and requests for interviews came from local and national media everywhere in the world. Whether community weeklies or large metropolitan dailies, all were interested in this story.

Mixed in with the calls from the media were quiet, hesitant inquiries from individuals who wanted to know what the procedure would involve, who would be eligible, and whom they might contact at the Clinic to register as possible candidates for the surgery.

Four years later, in December 2008, I lead the team that performed the first face transplant in the United States, making international headlines.

This book is a response to that attention. It's intended for those who may be interested in the evolution of a microsurgeon, those interested in the medicine that will allow a face transplant, those hoping for a new life, and those who contemplate giving hidden sufferers a new life and permission to walk in sunlight once again. I wanted to tell something of my life, not because it's particularly exciting or laden with adventure, but because it shows the path someone would follow en route to conducting a procedure that has never before been attempted.

I've been fortunate not only to be a surgeon but also to be an active researcher in transplantology, one who has made several contributions to the field. My fundamental role is to restore quality of life to those who have been deprived of it by disease or trauma. For me, as for all other transplant surgeons, test tubes, microscopes, and laboratory benches are as important as scalpels.

There are reasons that this transplant was not considered possible until the dawn of the 21st century. It's not because surgeons lacked the skills — those have existed for decades. The impediment to the procedure was our lack of understanding of the immune system and the concomitant inability to influence it. That impediment no longer stands. We can now manipulate the system, not perfectly and not with the finesse we would like, but sufficiently to prevent rejection of a composite-tissue allograft (tissue transplanted from another human): a face transplant.

At this time our understanding of the immune response is far from complete. I want to emphasize this point, especially to those readers and their friends who may be contemplating the procedure now or in the future. At present, all composite-tissue allograft transplants that involve different tissues require a lifelong commitment to a strict regimen of healthy living and immunosuppressive drugs. In this regard the patient is perhaps more responsible for the success of the procedure than all the medical specialists involved.

The purpose of this book is also to demonstrate the value of the gift to those who are considering becoming donors as well as to those who have yet to consider the idea. It is not an attempt to encourage donors to come forth. Rather it lays out the evidence for all to see: the history, labor, challenges, and need.

CHAPTER 1

Inching Ahead

ON JULY 15, 1410, in rolling green fields just outside the village of Grunwald, some 39,000 Poles and Lithuanians met and defeated 27,000 Teutonic knights and soldiers in what is said to have been the greatest battle of the Middle Ages. It is a struggle and triumph familiar to every citizen of Poland, but with the exception of a few history buffs and military historians, few outside the borders of my homeland seem to have heard of it.

The quiet, unpretentious neighborhood of Grunwald in Poznan, Poland, was named after that battle. This is the land of my youth.

Each day began with a bowl of warm milk soup, rolls spread with butter and cheese and sausage. This was plenty for a young girl on her way to school. I'd shoulder a big, square backpack known as a *tornister* and scamper down the steps to the street to start the half-hour walk to Elementary School 44. My friend Barbara would join me on the way, and we'd talk, giggle, and discuss our plans and dreams as we strolled past houses and small corner stores where portly, rosy-cheeked merchants sold fruit, candy, soda, beer, and newspapers.

Elementary School 44 was a monster. It needed to be big. In 1957, Poland was wrestling with the post–war baby boom. My classes held 40 or more children, and the school day was divided into morning and afternoon sessions to accommodate the crush.

The first few years of my education were dominated by Mrs. Dzierzkiewicz, who taught us grammar, reading, writing, mathematics, and art. Periodically she turned us loose in the tree-encircled playground outside.

Oh, how those trees and the sunlit playground called to me! As Mrs. Dzierzkiewicz talked about the role played by the Odra River in the nation's commerce, I'd imagine myself riding in the Tour de Pologne, a bicycle race that at the time began in Gdansk in the north and wound for more than 1,200 miles over hills and down through tree-filled valleys to Karpacz in the south. With the wind in my face and the sun on my shoulders, I flashed past cheering onlookers and sped across the finish line and back into reality, where barges laden with coal figured heavily in the development of industry in the communities along the banks of the river.

I did well academically from the day I entered elementary school until the day I received my degree from medical school. At the time, I didn't think I was especially gifted, but the truth is I loved to learn and loved to excel.

I left the *szkola podstawowa*, my elementary school, with a *swiadectwo ukonczenia szkoly podstawowej* (certificate of completion of primary school education) at age 14 and began my secondary education. In Poland, there is no equivalent of American middle schools.

My friend Barbara and I were fortunate to be accepted to Lyceum No. 2, a highly respected girls' school that proudly displayed its red number two on the dark blue uniforms we wore for the next four years.

Those years sped past. I remember our Russian teacher, a truly handsome man, tall with blue eyes. He always wore a suit, tie, and smile. He called us *panienki* (young ladies). That was a moment to remember. After all the candy and giggles and playgrounds and winning the Tour de Pologne during so many spring afternoon geography lessons, I had become a young lady — a lady!

Our uniforms were blue with white collars. You could

buy them at almost any clothing shop in Poznan, although some of the girls from families who were better off had their uniforms tailor-made. Tailor-made or off the rack, it didn't change much. Blue was still blue.

There was only one way we could assert our individuality. Although the dress code was very strict in specifying the uniform, its authors neglected to insert any legal language governing the color of stockings. That was our loophole. At the end of class periods the halls filled with rivers of young girls, all in blue, but wearing stockings that displayed every conceivable color and pattern in nature. My stockings were a dark green plaid. I was so proud the first day I wore them that I still smile at the thought of how I strutted.

I APPLIED FOR medical school during my last year at the Lyceum. I was drawn to the humanitarian aspect of studying medicine and the challenge to get accepted to medical school. My grades were good, but that was no guarantee of acceptance. Competition was tough, with a dozen applications for each opening.

The day came in early summer when a long and anxiously awaited list was posted by the dean's office. On it were the names of students who were accepted to the *Akademia Medyczna w Poznaniu* (Poznan University of

Medical Sciences). When you see your name on such a list, there's a fleeting moment of confusion and uncertainty before reality hits. There was my name! It was spelled correctly. It was most assuredly my name. I knew because I checked several times and then several times more. I was accepted. I was going to be a doctor.

A journey lay ahead that would take me through many countries, institutions, and patients' lives. At that time, I was an eager young woman, looking ahead to a future bright with possibilities. Now that I'm a recognized microsurgeon, I can see that the clinical path I followed was part of another path, one that stretches back 2,000 years.

ALL HISTORIANS OF transplant procedure feel obliged to note a Chinese physician named Pien Chi'ao. It is said that about 2,500 years ago he exchanged the heart of a man with a strong spirit but a weak will with the heart of a man who had a weak spirit but a strong will. This is a myth, of course, but the story has value. It shows that 2,500 years before the first true heart transplant was conducted, people were thinking that it was possible to use one individual's tissues and organs to restore another's.

It also illustrates the psychological attributes we attach to certain organs. The heart pumps blood. It is not the source of strong spirits or weak wills, but it makes for a good myth now as it did then. Even today, when heart transplants are common, we tend to give more emotional weight to certain organs and tissues than we do to others. The heart is one such organ. The tissues that compose the face are another.

An Indian surgeon named Susruta is credited with performing the first cosmetic surgery sometime between 1,000 and 600 BC. It was a practice at the time to slice the noses from criminals, as much to identify and humiliate them as to punish them. Susruta's skill lay in repairing the damage. Unlike Pien Chi'ao's mythical transplants, Susruta's undoubtedly took place, for he left concise instructions for his colleagues and successors. A reasonably experienced surgeon could follow the guidelines today. In the journal article "History of Plastic Surgery in India," R. E. Rana and B. S. Arora presented the guidelines:

The leaf of a creeper, long and broad enough to fully cover the whole of the severed or clipped off part, should be gathered. A patch of living flesh, equal in dimension to the preceding leaf, should be sliced off from the region of the cheek. After scarifying the severed nose with a knife, the flesh is swiftly adhered to it. Insert two small pipes in the nostrils to facilitate respiration and to prevent flesh from hanging down. The adhesioned part is dusted with the powders of Pattanga, Yashtimadhukam, and Rasanjana pulverized together. The nose should be enveloped in Karpasa cotton and several times sprinkled over with the refined oil of pure Sesamum. When the healing is complete and parts have united, remove the excess skin.

In AD 348, Saints Cosmas and Damian, the patrons of physicians and pharmacists, are said to have replaced the gangrenous leg of a Roman deacon with a leg removed from a recently deceased Ethiopian. Although this falls well into the realm of miracle and certainly wasn't possible according to what we now know about the immune system and tissue rejection, scholar Gabriel Meier noted that the event was portrayed in more than 1,500 paintings or illustrations. Apparently, several centuries before the invention of the printing press or the rise of mass media, the public was inspired by stunning medical feats.

Johannes Gutenberg perfected the first printing press by 1440. *De Curtorum Chirurgia per Insitionem* by Gaspare Tagliacozzi was published 57 years later. It's the first medical text to describe a tissue-transplant technique designed to restore noses mutilated by trauma or disease. Tagliacozzi, who practiced in Bologna at the close of the

16th century, was among the first to note the effects of an acute immunological response by observing that although an individual could receive and nurture his or her own transplanted flesh (an autograft), the transplanted flesh of another (an allograft) was invariably rejected. He also originated the nose job, and many credit him with being the father of cosmetic surgery.

The late 1500s were a violent, disease-ridden time. Noses were hacked and whacked in duels and in practices for duels. Noses were also disfigured by syphilis, a disease that had arrived in Italy about a century earlier.

Tagliacozzi's procedure involved cutting a flap of flesh from the forearm and fitting it into place over flesh removed from the nose. The flesh was left attached to the arm to ensure reliable blood flow to the tissue while it grew into place on the nose. The doctor devised an elaborate structure to hold the arm to the nose for about two weeks. When the arm's flesh had healed to the nose, the flap was cut loose and the patient was free to move into society with a reconstructed nose.

The procedure was conducted long before the creation of anesthetics, so it must be concluded that the doctor's patients were exceedingly motivated to restore their looks, since they willingly suffered what must have been a terribly painful procedure.

Tagliacozzi also has the dubious credit of being one of the first cosmetic surgeons to awaken a stormy ethical discussion in society — or at least that part of society that was represented by the Church. At the beginning of the Renaissance, although many mutilated noses resulted from war or legal procedures (the law allowed for noses to be removed from thieves and other miscreants), most traumatized noses had been disfigured by syphilis. Church authorities appear to have taken the position that God punished people for sexual transgressions by marking them for all to see. Legal authorities thought the idea had merit, and subsequently noses were lopped from the faces of a variety of miscreants. The Church reasoned that anyone attempting to restore a nose to its former condition was attempting to circumvent either church law or God's will. Either action carried consequences. The belief that disease and disfigurement represent the actions of a higher power, one whose decisions should not be tampered with, continues to be held by a number of religious sects today.

On June 4, 1894, Marie François Sadi Carnot, the president of France, had finished giving a speech at a banquet in Lyon and was settling into the seat of an open carriage when the Italian anarchist Sante Caserio elbowed aside the top-hatted dignitaries, leaped into the carriage, and plunged a dagger into the president's abdomen. The blade severed the portal vein, which carries blood from the intestine to the liver. Surgeons tried but lacked the skill to repair the damaged vein, and the president died within hours.

Twenty-one-year-old Alexis Carrel, then a medical student at the University of Lyon, took note and resolved that no patient in his care would die because his skills were insufficient to the challenge.

Carrel, a diminutive man with one brown eye and one blue, turned to Madame Leroudier, reputed to be the finest seamstress in the city. Few in the world matched her skills at embroidery and needlepoint. It is said that when he finished studying her technique with fine needles and threads, he could join two edges of paper together with not a stitch showing on either side.

One observer, remarking upon Carrel's skills, said that he could join blood vessels "as small as a matchstick." A standard household matchstick is roughly 2.5 to 3 millimeters in diameter. (A "hair's breadth" is 0.0039 inch. A microsurgical needle can be as small as 0.00196 inches, almost exactly half a hair's breadth.) The vessels and nerves being joined today have diameters less than 1 mm, about the size of the lead in a mechanical pencil.

A significant part of the challenge facing the young

doctor was maintaining the structural integrity of diminutive vessels during anastomosis (attaching one tube to another) and preserving it afterward. It's nearly impossible to sew one end of a tiny, slippery vessel to another and get both tubes properly aligned and stable when the vessels are unanchored. Imagine trying to sew the ends of two pieces of spaghetti together when they are resting on a wet plate.

Surgeons would stabilize the vessels by placing temporary sutures on each side and anchoring them to nearby anatomy, much as one would stabilize a rowboat by tying it between two docks. However, when tension was placed on the two sutures, the end of the vessel would be distorted to the shape of a squinting eye.

Carrel improved on this by placing three sutures at equal distances (120 degrees) around the vessel. When the sutures were tightened, the vessel's opening would assume the shape of a triangle. The opposite vessel was anchored and distorted to the same shape, allowing the triangular ends of the vessels to be matched accurately and then sutured.

Dr. Carrel was looking farther into the future than perhaps he knew. It would be years before tissues and organs could be transplanted with any degree of consistency, but the obstacle was no longer technical. Dr. Carrel had shown conclusively that human skill and well-practiced technique were sufficient to the task.

The modern era of plastic and reconstructive surgery can be traced to a day in 1917 when Dr. Harold Gillies walked into the operating room of what was then called The Queen's Hospital in Sidcup, a district in London. The First World War had been killing men or mutilating their bodies for nearly three years. In previous wars, an operation was thought to be successful if it saved a man's life. Dr. Gillies felt that surgeons' skills should restore form as well as function to the men who were wounded. He argued for and won the establishment of the 1,000-bed Queens Hospital, a facility dedicated to the wholly new specialty of plastic surgery. During the course of the war, he and his colleagues would perform more than 11,000 surgeries on 5,000 men.

Some of these were successful beyond all medical experience to date. Some weren't. In an excellent article on World War I and facial disfigurement published in the February 2007 issue of *Smithsonian* magazine, Caroline Alexander describes the impact of the war on soldiers' faces:

> *Those patients who could be successfully treated were, after lengthy convalescence, sent on their way; the less fortunate remained in hospitals and conva-*

lescent units nursing the broken faces with which they were unprepared to confront the world — or with which the world was unprepared to confront them. In Sidcup...some park benches were painted blue, a code that warned townspeople that any man sitting on one of them would be distressful to view. A more upsetting encounter, however, was often between the disfigured man and his own image. Mirrors were banned in most wards...

In the years between the World Wars, as men and women sought cosmetic surgical procedures to alter unattractive but otherwise acceptable features, a host of critics railed against the procedures as unnecessary exercises in vanity and attempts to circumvent the work of God. Their arguments were similar to those directed at Tagliacozzi in 15th-century Italy.

But the critics failed to dampen enthusiasm for the new cosmetic treatments that by the 1920s had acquired an aura of sophistication. In 1924, the *New York Daily Mirror* held a contest to "take the homeliest girl in the biggest city in the country and make a beauty of her." Today, the equivalent of that newspaper contest can be found in such television shows as *Extreme Makeover.* The only thing missing is the controversy.

While these procedures advanced the surgical techniques associated with transplant procedures, each involved the patient's own tissue and bone. Although allografts were no doubt attempted on occasion, tissue from any source other than the recipient was invariably rejected. The obstacle presented by the immune system remained unmoved.

In the early 1930s, the Russian surgeon Yuriy Yurievich Voronoy challenged the system when he made several attempts to transplant kidneys from cadavers to patients in need. All attempts failed, and his patients died. His efforts did not advance the science of transplants but did earn him a lasting place in texts on medical ethics.

By 1939, it was understood that certain blood groups were incompatible, that certain cells released proteins called antibodies, and that these antibodies fought both disease and foreign tissue. A handful of researchers and physicians thought that other cells, such as phagocytes, had a role in immunity, but their views were not widely held.

In September 1939, Hitler's armies invaded my homeland. During and after World War II, the world's politics, science, medicine, and technologies have changed rapidly and radically. The concept of total war meant targeting both troops and civilian centers with high explosives and incendiary bombs. Hospitals were overwhelmed with military and civilian casualties. Physicians became fairly proficient with autografts, but in many patients, particularly those who were severely burned, there was not enough healthy, undamaged tissue to be transplanted.

The British Medical Council assigned a young zoologist named Peter Medawar to study the problem. Dr. Medawar reported what many others had observed but had failed to shape into a comprehensive overview of transplant rejection. Dr. Medawar noted that while autografts succeeded, tissue transplanted from others was invariably rejected, even when such tissue seemed to have been accepted initially. Moreover, subsequent allografts were rejected nearly immediately. The conclusion to be drawn was that transplant recipients had been immunized to foreign tissue by the initial transplant.

The war also brought advances in anesthesiology that permitted longer and more extensive procedures. The first antibiotics reduced the loss of transplant to infection. One of the more discouraging events affecting surgeons and patients was to have the success of a lengthy transplant operation eradicated by an opportunistic microbe in the days following the procedure.

In the 1950s, the surgical world turned again. A number of elements came together to create what would become one of the more important decades in the history of transplants.

In 1954 Dr. Joseph Murray entered an operating room at Peter Bent Brigham Hospital in Boston, Massachusetts, and transplanted a kidney from one twin to another. The organ was accepted, and both twins survived. The reason would eventually be explained in research conducted by Jean Dausset, head of the Immunohematology Laboratory at France's National Blood Transfusion Center, who described the first histocompatibility antigen. This was one of a set of genes in the major histocompatibility complex (MHC) that produce the cell-surface proteins that allow the immune system to differentiate between self-tissue and foreign tissue. As might be suspected, they play a major role in determining whether transplanted tissue will be accepted or rejected. The sibling who received the transplant survived because the twins were identical. The identifying protein manufactured in one twin's MHC matched perfectly that of the other twin.

Still, there are only so many identical twins. In 1959 Robert Schwartz and William Dameshek at the Tufts University School of Medicine, Boston, identified a substance called 6-mercaptopurine. A derivative of this drug known as azathioprine (Imuran, Azasan) suppressed the immune system. The drug's ability to inhibit transplant rejection opened the world of transplant procedures.

The holy grail of transplant procedures was less than ten years away.

On December 3, 1967, in an operating room in Groote Schuur Hospital, Cape Town, South Africa, Dr. Christiaan Barnard took the heart out of Denise Darvall, a young woman who suffered irreversible brain damage in a car accident, and put it into the chest of a 55-year-old grocer named Louis Washkansky. Mr. Washkansky died 18 days later of pneumonia. He had been left vulnerable to the disease by heavy doses of drugs meant to suppress his immune responses to Miss Darvall's heart.

By the close of the 1960s, more than 100 heart transplants had been conducted, but the procedure had an 85 percent mortality rate primarily due to tissue rejection. Surgeons had mastered the technical challenges. The immune system remained a barrier.

The barrier would be surmounted in the 1970s when Swiss biologist Jean-François Borel isolated a compound from *Beauvaria nivea*, a fungus that had been collected in Wisconsin and at Norway's Hardangervidda by traveling employees of Sandoz, a Swiss pharmaceutical company. The Hardangervidda is a windswept and treeless plateau said to be inhabited only by reindeer, grasses, lichens, mosses, and life-saving fungi. Sandoz, like many other such companies, had a program that routinely screened organic compounds from around the world for biological activity. The initial studies of the compounds drawn from the fungi showed them to have some immunosuppressive properties, but little else.

At the time, the market for immunosuppressive drugs was small because so few transplant procedures were being conducted. If not for the persistence of Dr. Borel and some of his associates, the curious fungus might have wound up as no more than a sheaf of yellowing pages of biological data with the term *fungal extract 24-556* somewhere on the cover page. When they analyzed and tested the compound against blood cells, they found it would inhibit only T-cells, the primary cells involved in graft rejection. Dr. Borel described the results as "too beautiful to be true." It was decided that fungal extract 24-556 would be called cyclosporin, a name now well known as the drug that revolutionized the field of transplant surgery and saved countless lives.

There would be refinements to immunosuppressive therapy in the coming years, but at this point the only parameters limiting transplant procedures were experience, skill, and technology. The century closed with a string of firsts. Among these were the first heart-lung transplant (1981), the first heart-liver transplant (1984), the first double lung transplant (1986), and the first sciatic nerve transplant (1988).

In 1998, Dr. Marshall Strome led a team of doctors at Cleveland Clinic in the first total larynx transplant. Three days after the surgery, forty-year-old patient Timothy Heidler spoke for the first time in 30 years. The first successful hand transplant was performed in Lyon, France, that same year.

Six years later, in 2004, based on my 20 years of research, Cleveland Clinic's Institutional Review Board granted the world's first approval to perform face transplants in humans.

CHAPTER 2

Anatomy Lessons

EVERY PROFESSION HAS an associated aroma. For auto mechanics, it's the smell of oil. For carpenters, it's sawdust. For medical students, it's formaldehyde — and it can be overpowering at age eighteen when you get your first whiff.

There's no such thing as "pre-med" in Poland. Students determine a career path early in their lives, going straight from high school into advanced study of their chosen professions. This means that students dreaming of someday being doctors go straight from high school to medical school, to anatomy labs and formaldehyde-soaked cadavers, before their 19th birthday.

Anatomy was one of the greater challenges young students faced in Poland. It was a hurdle that had to be leapt in at least three languages: Polish, Russian, and Latin, the universal language of medicine. At the *Akademia Medyczna w Poznaniu*, anatomy classes were offered in two buildings on Swiecicki Street. One contained one of the largest auditoriums in the medical school, a cavernous room easily able to hold the 200-plus students taking the class. The texts and reference works for the class consisted of 12 volumes of illustrations and text in Polish by Drs. Adam Bochenek and Michal Reicher. It's one of the few medical works in continuous print for nearly a century.

The material was horribly compressed, the illustrations were small, and the labels identifying the various aspects of organs were even smaller. It was difficult to link the organ in the illustration with the corresponding organ in a body. Today students have videotapes of operations and dissections, and can turn to their computers to rotate an organ through three dimensions. The best we could do with Bochenek and Reicher to get another viewpoint was to turn the book upside down. It's surprising that so many medical students graduated with their eyesight intact.

There was also a three-volume atlas of anatomy in Russian that served as a backup text for the Bochenek and Reicher volumes. The lecture absorbed two to three hours a day, every day, and the usual reading assignment from one day to the next was 150 pages. Our professors, as sadistic as most other medical school professors, would ask questions derived from not only the body of the text but the fine print as well.

I don't think that any student in the class got a grade higher than "C" during the first weeks of the class. Not only didn't we know anatomy, we didn't know how to study anatomy. We learned both. It's not as if we had a choice.

After the lecture, 20 of us would troop next door to the Collegium Anatomicum; don caps, gowns, and gloves; pick up scalpels; and march somewhat hesitantly into the rooms that held the cadavers. The reek of formaldehyde was strong enough to induce vertigo.

It would be inaccurate to call the bodies lying on display cadavers. They were the phantoms of cadavers. Cadavers were expensive, so the school tended to use them until their organs completely lost any instructive or informative value. The chest cavities were open and internal organs lay in place, although they had already been separated, or presected, in preparation for anatomy class from the body by a skilled anatomist. The instructor would lift an organ and begin asking questions: Where were the primary arteries? The primary veins? How would the organ be oriented if it were still in place? What is this? Where would one expect to find that? What is the function of this?

The students greeted these initial lessons with bad jokes. We were 18 or 19 years old, rather young to be reaching into a body cavity to pick up a liver, handle a lung, or trace the path that nerves weave as they move from the arm through muscle and tendon to the shoulder and into the brain. I suppose it could be called graveyard humor, although it's probably more accurately described as anatomy-lab humor, and I suspect it's found in every medical school in the world. It was understandable. We were thrown into some very deep waters.

As the class progressed, the jokes eventually stopped. I don't know whether it was our age or the nature of the class, but we matured substantially that semester as our respect for the complexity of human anatomy grew.

Although there were only 10 students to a cadaver, there were at least 220 students rotating through anatomy studies each semester, and the unfortunate cadavers began to show signs of wear. Some of the organs on display in the local butcher shop were more recognizable than those we were studying.

Classes and cadavers were not our only source of anatomical information. The lecture hall and classrooms held all variety of diseased organs on display in formaldehyde-filled glass jars. It was a chance for students to see how cancer progresses through a lung or the effects of diabetes on a kidney. Although the cadaver spread on the table in the Collegium was much closer to a person than were the diseased organs and tissues floating in the jars, those were more disturbing. It was startling to see how much damage disease could cause in an organ that is vital to life. We knew what kidneys and other organs were supposed to look like and where they should be. They looked very out of place in a jar in a lecture hall. It bothered me for the entire year.

The class and cadaver study were merely an introduction to anatomy, a sort of formaldehyde-soaked overview. The real study of anatomy begins when a young surgeon scrubs in with a more experienced surgeon. Sooner or later the experienced surgeon will tell his young protégé to pick up a scalpel or ask that sutures be placed there, there, and there. This is the beginning of the true study of anatomy, because it's not about the names of things or their locations, but the resistance different tissues offer to blades and needles. It's about the caution necessary during dissection because of the tendency of veins to hide behind this or nerves to run through that. It's about how slippery tissues and vessels can be when they're wearing a coat of blood, and it's about how much patience and perseverance is needed to join the opposing ends of a vessel severed by an ax.

MY EXPLORATION OF anatomy began with those thin cadavers in the Collegium and progressed as I began to scrub in on general surgeries. It would progress further when I decided to specialize in orthopedic procedures, and when in Finland and Louisville, Kentucky, I came to a focus and began to study the hand. These studies led me to consider the possibility of a face transplant and to work toward that goal.

Many of the hand procedures my colleagues and I completed involved patients whose hands had been burned in accidents. Some of these burns were extensive and facial disfigurement was not unusual. The hands, when scarred by trauma and numerous repairs, can always be enclosed in gloves. When the face suffers similar misfortune, the patient has the choice of displaying the disfigurement to the world or hiding in the shadows. Far too many choose the latter.

I hoped to change that.

NO OTHER ANATOMICAL structure compares in complexity to the face. The hand approximates it. Some would argue that the complexity of the hand equals that of the face, but although the hand may have more obvious parts, the face has a more intricate, complicated, and subtle musculature.

Lie down and rest a wet handkerchief over your face. It will conform to the structure that lies beneath, even if it's someone else's handkerchief. We expect the face taken from the donor and placed upon the recipient to do the same.

Nerves bring impulse to the face muscles, telling them when to pucker, when to spit, and when to squint. These nerves also penetrate the skin to a point near the surface, allowing it to register heat, cold, pressure, and pain.

The face can be divided into three broad plateaus. The ophthalmic plane covers the forehead, eyes, and nose. The maxillary plane starts above the temples and covers the cheeks and sides of the nose. The mandibular plane also starts above the temples and covers the lower jaw and chin. The nerves that run into these three planes branch like the limbs of a willow tree from the trigeminal nerve, which lies beneath the parotid gland, the largest of the salivary glands. This gland lies just beneath the ear at the back of the jaw.

Place your finger at the corner of your eye and trace a line back to the tragus, the small bit of flesh that protrudes into the ear's canal. Move your finger forward and down an inch or so, and it will be resting above the trigeminal nerve at about the point where it branches to reach the three plateaus of the face. This is primarily a sensory nerve. Signals from a bang on the head to a drop of rain to a toothache will travel along one of the many branches of this nerve.

The motor impulses that generate expressions travel along the facial nerve. Move your finger from the tragus down to a spot just beneath the bottom tip of the ear. Your finger will be resting on or near the facial nerve. This nerve carries signals from the brain to the muscles of the face that express emotion. A semi-rare disease called Bell's palsy results from an ear inflammation that puts pressure on the nerve, leading to paralysis of half the face. A rare congenital condition is the absence of the facial nerve, a loss that prohibits an individual from registering any facial emotion or expression. The neurologists who describe this condition note that it has severe social consequences.

If your finger is still beneath your ear, draw it straight down the side of your neck and stop just before you reach the collarbone. If your fingers are resting lightly on the side of your neck, you should feel the throb of blood flowing through the carotid artery, the primary conduit of blood to every cell in the face. The jugular vein lies beneath it to return blood from the artery's many branches back to the heart.

These are the primary vessels that will feed and drain a facial allograft. They will be connected to the transplant before the recipient's face is removed, allowing us to determine whether the transplant is feasible. If transplanted tissue does not fill and drain properly (i.e., pink up), it will not be used, the patient's vessels will be reconnected, and his or her face will be retained.

The need to match artery to artery, vein to vein, and nerve to nerve is what sets the face transplant apart from a standard facial tissue transplant. Tissue transplants that are used to restore some semblance of normalcy to a disfigured face involve taking thin sections of skin from elsewhere on a patient's body. For many victims of severe burns, recovering patches that will cover more than a small portion of the face is impossible.

Even in disfigured patients whose bodies may be whole, acquiring enough tissue to cover a face in its entirety may be impossible. We have learned from cadaver studies that the mean surface area covered by facial tissue can be as large as 184 square inches. This is more than a square foot of flesh. Even if this much tissue were available, say from a back, abdomen, or thigh, it would be nothing like facial tissue. It would not be nearly so pliable and it would have to be forced to conform to underlying structures and anatomy.

It would be a cardboard mask.

The more you know about anatomy, the more you realize there's still more to learn. The experience might be compared to a move to a new city. For a long time you need a map to find your way around, but after several years of experience the boulevards, streets, and alleys become known and, as the saying goes, are as familiar as the back of your hand. Still, as I would discover, few subjects in anatomy are as complex as the hand or face.

CHAPTER 3

Wanderings

THE SOUNDS OF guitars, violins, and accordions drifted across the outdoor café. Dark-haired musicians in festive dress circled our table of giggling young women, eyes flashing as they played, winking and grinning as if they knew secrets about us that we didn't know ourselves.

The first time the burden of intensive study was lifted, the first time I was truly away from home on my own, came during the fall of my third year of medical school when my friends and I vacationed for two weeks at Lake Balaton in western Hungary. Natives of Poland, Hungary, and other nations of central Europe who have been to Lake Balaton know the moonlight, the songs, the wines, and the small cafés that grace its shores. In

Hungary, a landlocked country, Lake Balaton is thought of as the nation's Mediterranean.

The lake is 50 miles long and 10 miles across at its widest point, circled by villages that dot the winding roads like bright beads on a string. Each small town is unique; each community prides itself on offering a landmark — a church, castle, or fine hotel — that its neighbors do not have.

During the day we wandered from the shore into the hills to visit the little towns, sit at outdoor cafés, and sample the local wines. Well-ordered vineyards dappled the surrounding hills, and the townspeople regarded their vintages as they did their firstborn children. (We fancied that we could almost hear each town whisper to its neighbors, "Your child is smart but let's face it, mine is much smarter. Please don't take it personally.") From this region came wines such as Szurkebarat, Keknyelu, Olaszrizling, Rizlingszilvani, Ottonel Muskotaly, Tramini, and the memorable Cserszegi Fuszeres ("spicy wine of Cserszeg"), a winner of many international awards.

To the crowd of young students wandering from café to café, sitting and watching the colored lights dance over the lake's dark waves and listening as the musicians played, every wine was special. Every evening, each vintage we sampled was the best we had ever tasted.

I returned to my classes refreshed. But I knew I had to get away again soon. When the following summer arrived after a winter's work, I found myself walking the canal-bordered streets of Genk, an industrial city of 60,000 in Flanders in western Belgium. Like many Belgian communities the city is crossed with canals that once served as boulevards for barges, boats, and ships laden with spices, silks, and exotic goods from around the world.

It was what might be called a working vacation. For a small fee, I was allowed to live in the nurses' quarters of Ziekenhuis Oost-Limburg. For three months, I was a nurse's aide, assisting the hospital's nurses and doctors. I was apprenticed to Dr. William DeVriews, and followed him on rounds, changed dressings, and assisted in the emergency room. He was a talented general surgeon who seemed able to do anything.

One afternoon a young man who had been in an accident was brought to the emergency room. Among his other injuries, his face bore a number of cuts, none serious, but substantial enough to merit sutures. The doctor tended him, then turned to me and said, "Sew him up."

These were the first of the thousands of sutures I would place during my professional life, but I remember them as if I did them this morning. A few days later the doctor, with me in tow, was making rounds and entered the young man's room to change his dressings. The doctor gently pulled the white gauze from the man's face and looked at the stitches, which I must say were wonderfully even. He nodded and said, "That is a very good job. Someday the young lady may become a good surgeon." I can't remember anything else that happened that day. I don't need to.

I wasn't the only such aide in the hospital. Young men and women from all over Europe apprenticed themselves to physicians or institutions in order to gain experience, build a network of new friends in the profession, and work where their weekends could be spent in outdoor cafés located as far from their hometowns as possible.

The Flemish countryside was speckled with small villages, one of which was home to friends of my relatives. On several occasions they invited me to spend the weekend and I readily accepted. The small houses in villages off the beaten tourist track are immaculately kept. They're 100 or 200 years old — some even older — but all look as if they've just been taken out of a box, scrubbed, and placed just so for the delight of passersby.

Many of these homes had large bay windows that looked onto the street. Their window boxes were filled with well-tended flowers, and the windows framed great displays of flowers arranged in a way that allowed those passing on the street to see the interior of the dwelling and its furnishings. As I passed these houses, it occurred to me that these displays of flowers and furniture were not presented solely to entertain visitors but also to demonstrate the taste and material success of the occupants. In America, they park a new car in the driveway. In Belgium, they put flowers in the window.

The summer also offered the opportunity to visit museums in Brugge, Antwerp, Brussels, and elsewhere that held the treasures of Dutch and Flemish art. Rubens's magnificent *Elevation of the Cross,* depicting muscled Romans and slaves lifting Jesus and the cross, stands above the altar in Antwerp's Our Lady's Cathedral. In the Netherlands I saw Rembrandt's *The Anatomy Lesson of Dr. Nicolaes Tulp* at the Mauritshuis Museum in The Hague. I was so taken by the painting's beauty, composition, and anatomical accuracy that a reproduction hangs in my Cleveland Clinic office today.

Art draws me away from the professional world, away from the sound of sirens and footsteps racing to emergency rooms, away from the concentration required to join severed arteries and the uncomprehending looks of patients who must be told that some, but not all, of a limb had been saved.

MY FIFTH YEAR of medical school found me in Barcelona. The hospitals of Europe offered an exchange program for medical students in which two students from Germany would be swapped for two from England, two promising young French urologists traded for a pair of family practitioners from Spain, and so on. The idea was to expose students to different experts, patterns of practice, cultures, and languages. It worked. I think doctors trained in this manner have a completely different worldview from those who have trained in only one or two institutions.

One morning as the summer was about to begin, I wrestled my suitcase aboard a train in Poznan. I was off to Barcelona, with a one-day layover in Paris.

The train slipped through the night, slowed, and crept into the cavernous Gare du Nord station in north Paris the next morning. There I was with a heavy suitcase, ten dollars in my pocket, and a long day ahead before I could board my connecting train at a station in the south of the city. It was to be a good day, a good day indeed.

That morning the great station echoed with the babble of foreign languages as travelers from all over Europe bustled through, coming from here, going there, hurrying to their connections. It was Paris. It was the beginning of summer. The station was awash with young people from Italy, England, Sweden, Belgium, Norway, and Germany.

Among them were two young men, medical students from San Francisco. Like all Americans, they were friendly, happy, talkative, and generous. At the station café I enjoyed a breakfast croissant and café au lait with these energetic Yankees, who spoke a brisk and happy form of English that I'd never heard before. When the cups were empty and set on the table for the last time, we did what every young person does in Paris when the only thing to worry about is catching an evening train. We walked and walked and walked, because, after all, it was Paris.

I had lunch with my new friends. We ate in a small café at the foot of Montmartre, the highest hill in Paris. Broad steps swarming with tourists led from the base of the hill up to the Sacré-Coeur Basilica, one of the more distinguished cathedrals in a city known for them. Many came to see the art and watch the sidewalk artists, who seemed to have been distributed at a ratio of roughly one artist for every four tourists.

The artists present that day came to Montmartre to paint because yesterday's artists had come there to paint. For this custom, Napoleon is responsible. When he came to power he wanted Paris redesigned, and the project drove many of the poorer inhabitants of the city's center to outlying communities, one of which was Montmartre. The area soon gained a reputation for good, inexpensive wine and all that follows good, inexpensive wine: conversation, laughter, music, more conversation. The area became home to actors, writers, poets, and artists.

I don't believe there is another spot on the planet that has felt the tread of so much genius: Camille Pissarro, Pablo Picasso, Amedeo Modigliani, Vincent van Gogh, Jacques Villon, Raymond Duchamp-Villon, Henri Matisse, Suzanne Valadon, Pierre-Auguste Renoir, Edgar Degas, Maurice Utrillo, and Henri de Toulouse-Lautrec, who immortalized the boozy patrons of the Moulin Rouge, a café in the red-light district that bordered Montmartre — all had been here.

When I bid farewell to the two future doctors from America, little did I know that I would one day be their colleague, a surgeon at one of the foremost hospitals in the United States.

The next morning, after another train ride through the night, I dragged my luggage along the Calle Casanova in Barcelona on my way to the city's University Hospital. For the next three months, I lived in the four-to-a-room single-nurses' quarters while I studied general surgery in the *Hospital Clinico i Provincial de Barcelona*. I passed many happy hours laughing and gabbing with nurses, medical students, and young doctors from all over the world at Tasko, the café across the street from the hospital. Every hospital in the world has a café, bar, diner, or cheap restaurant across the street that serves as a hangout for young people in medicine. There must be a zoning law requiring it.

The café was always full of laughter, talk, smoke, and the sound of clinking glasses filled with rum and Coke, the drink of the moment. The students exchanged stories of the day's medical events, what this doctor had done, what that doctor hadn't, what a curious case this patient was, and places you had to visit in Barcelona.

La Rambla is a mile-long boulevard running through the heart of the city's center. Closed to traffic, it's flanked by great trees that cast islands of shadow on the wide promenade and teems with flower stalls, cafés, art shops, trinket sellers, dancers, mimes, and musicians. If you could choose any place in the world to sit in a café and watch the people of the world pass by, La Rambla would be it.

Sometimes you meet someone and you just know you are going to be friends. I met Sirkka Liukkonen in Barcelona. She was studying obstetrics and gynecology, and together we traveled Spain, or as much of it as we could get to on the few weekends we had off. Sirkka and I joined three students from France who had a Citroën.

We would crowd into the old car, count our change so we could share the cost of gas, and be off through the night, rambling and bumping along Spain's country roads to the music of Jethro Tull and Pink Floyd.

We followed the twisting roads north to Figueras to visit Salvador Dalí's home and museum, drove south along the coast road, and sometimes ventured into the mountainous interior, where every dusty town seemed to have its own castle. If you come to know a country by following a carefully chosen path, you're on a tour. If you chase after an idea that you wake up with in the morning, you're on an adventure. Young medical students burdened throughout the week with work and study aren't interested in tours.

I returned to the hospital the next year with two Polish friends to study surgery. We had gathered in Barcelona's harbor to catch a ferry to Majorca, the largest of the three Balearic Islands off Spain's eastern coast in the Mediterranean. The sun was setting. The ferry would not leave until the morning. We had enough money for fruit and coffee, but none for lodging. This set of circumstances was so familiar that we thought little of it, applied our imaginations, and decided to spend the night camped amid large stores of timber waiting for shipment to who knows where.

Enter Sergeant Garcia. In 1974 Spain still belonged to the dictator Generalissimo Francisco Franco and his fascist minions, one of whom — well fed, well armed, and in uniform — confronted us three Polish medical students camped in a pile of lumber. We immediately dubbed him "Sergeant Garcia" due to his striking resemblance to the bumbling, officious Mexican soldier whose principal duty was to offer comic relief on the *Zorro* television show.

I was the only one of us who spoke Spanish, and although it took some doing, I managed to convince him that we were neither stealing lumber nor bent on the overthrow of the nation. That I was twenty years old and blue-eyed with flowing blond hair may have helped.

The next day we moved through the rooms of the grand stone Carthusian monastery on Majorca where another Pole, Frédéric Chopin, and his mistress, George Sand, spent the cold, damp winter of 1838–39. There, in a small room, stood the humble upright piano on which Chopin composed *Les Preludes*. One of the monastery's caretakers has the melancholy task of placing a single rose on the keyboard every morning. After visiting the homes and hangouts of so many artists throughout Europe, I found that it gave me an odd feeling to come to this windy island so far off the coast of Spain and find home by reading Chopin's letters written in Polish.

Chopin died of consumption, otherwise known as pulmonary tuberculosis, ten years after that winter sojourn. The disease is eminently curable today, and it's worth wondering how much more great music he might have given the world had the intervention of modern medicine been possible.

Medicine is a universal language for my colleagues and me. In my youth, when I first left Poland for the rest of the world, I have to confess that I had something of an inferiority complex. I was, after all, from a country that had suffered heavily during World War II, then suffered again as a satellite socialist nation. My fears were dispelled quickly at the clinics, emergency rooms, operating theaters, and patient bedsides where I learned that the medical skills I had acquired from my teachers in Poland were as good as any acquired by my foreign colleagues. In some instances, they were better.

Whether I was in Belgium or Spain, when I met foreign colleagues, we spoke medicine and understood each other quite well. More than 30 years later, I still find myself on the streets of foreign cities, bumping into colleagues and speaking medicine. It's a great language, and it's a privilege to be able to speak it.

౷

CHAPTER 4

Of Scalpels and Family

IT'S SAFE TO assume that when the bright green John Deere 4020 powershift tractor rolled off the assembly line in Waterloo, Iowa, sometime in 1963, none of the machine's designers ever said, "Gee, maybe we ought to have the owner's manual translated into Polish." This understandable oversight got me a job that helped me through medical school and led to my marriage.

The Biuro Tlumaczy (Bureau of Translation) was on the second floor of an Art Deco building in Poznan. At the top of the stairs, one entered a room with a great high ceiling lit in the afternoon by sunlight flooding through equally tall windows. Behind a counter stood a row of desks. One was for the bureau's lawyer, who was essential to the work of the office because of the large number of documents filled with English, German, Spanish, French, or Russian legalese needing translation into Polish legalese. Another desk was occupied by the translation manager, who passed out assignments to the appropriate specialists, one of whom was me.

I was fluent in English and was able to pick up extra money for my education, ice cream, and theater tickets by translating all manner of documents from English to Polish. These included medical and pharmacological papers on diseases and treatments. I also worked on nonscientific papers, private letters, and owner/operator manuals for tractors, cultivators, corn harvesters, and other farm equipment. Within a few years I'd be in Kentucky suturing hands and fingers back onto men who probably should have paid closer attention to exactly such manuals.

Much of the work was boring, but the walk to the bureau to pick up the material was pleasant, especially after several hours spent at a medical lecture. Poznan, like all old central European cities, has acquired a wealth of architecture through the centuries. Each passing monarch, successful merchant, or dominant politician established a place in history by building an edifice reflecting the architectural influences of the time. During the spring and autumn, the 20-minute walk took me past buildings whose façades reflected centuries of changing architectural fads and fashions.

As I walked, I tried not to be distracted by all the bookstalls, cafés, and fashions in the shop windows. To complete that trip on a warm spring afternoon without stopping was a challenge to anyone's self-discipline and meager budget.

Sometimes I'd pick up an assignment and instead of returning home to work, I'd find an empty desk at the bureau, spread out my pencils, paper, and dictionaries, and begin to translate. I was equally familiar with English and Polish terminology for all aspects of medical and biological science, but the terms for the components of snapping rollers, husking beds, and corn delivery augers sometimes exceeded my vocabulary.

I called for help and got it in the form of a handsome young man named Wlodzimierz. We spent several hours arguing about the nomenclature of corn-picker parts and the correct grammar for instructions detailing their assembly, maintenance, and operation. Then we found that we had more in common than an ability to translate obscure English terms into equally obscure Polish terms. We liked movies. We liked music. We liked each other. We were married in the chapel at the city's town hall on April 27, 1975. I wore light blue.

I suspect that many Americans must think that getting married at a town hall is a somewhat pedestrian way for two people to begin a new life. They're imagining the sort of granite-and-glass town halls that hunker in the center of American cities like bureaucratic fortresses.

But Poznan's town hall was built 700 years ago at the turn of the 13th century. It burned in 1536 and was rebuilt by the Italian architect Giovanni Battista di Quadro, who created what was said to be the most beautiful structure north of the Alps. Over the next 500 years, fires, gales, lightning strikes, and wars led to cycles of destruction, rebuilding, and restoration. The face of the building that now looks into the town square consists of three colonnaded arcades, rising one atop the other like the layers of a great cake. The arcades are surmounted by three towers, one at each corner and one in the center bearing a clock.

Renaissance architects had a remarkable ability to fuse beauty, practicality, and humor. Every day at noon, two mechanical billy goats emerge from beneath the clock to inform the citizens of the town that the day has reached midpoint.

On a warm day in April, under a sunny blue sky, with the cobblestone square bustling with citizens anticipating spring and the billy goats nestled in their tower awaiting their midday duties, there is no more romantic place in Poland to get married than the chapel in Poznan Town Hall. Did I mention that I wore blue?

ONE OF THE MAJOR differences between falling in love and practicing medicine is that the former does not require a great deal of research. And for the most part, being in love is usually more exciting than research — but not always.

Like love, research involves imagination and a certain amount of daydreaming. Researchers dream of the "elegant" experiment, a decided rarity. An elegant experiment is one that is designed so simply, so logically, and so tightly that its results cannot be challenged. Elegant research, or an elegant experiment, makes the resultant data seem obvious. The findings derived from such experiments are unquestionably true, and with luck the results add something valuable to the sum of our medical understanding of health and disease.

It would seem that designing an elegant experiment or research project would be simple. Take someone with health problem "A," give him compound "B," and see what happens ("C"). While this sort of experiment seems simple, it's contaminated with dozens, even hundreds, of known and unknown variables. Researchers have a profound dislike for known and unknown variables that borders on paranoia.

A good piece of research or a well-designed experiment takes into account the known variables and either eliminates them, reduces them to a negligible and measurable impact, or adjusts for them in one manner or another.

An unknown variable, one that appears unexpectedly at the end of an experiment — or, worse yet, one that is identified by a colleague at another institution when the study is being reviewed for publication — can send months, even years of painstaking work into the toxic-waste bin at the far end of the laboratory.

When elegance is impossible, researchers strive for the sort of experimental design that accounts for all variables and produces data that may not answer all questions, yet answers enough to advance the field and allow new, more promising questions to be asked. The value of the answer depends on how well the question is framed, so we're extremely careful when doing so.

Patience, precision, and careful analysis: these are the qualities of research I first began to learn in the laboratories of Dr. Jadwiga Przedpelska, a slender, petite woman with gray hair always tightly held back by a black bow. She spoke slowly in a thin, high voice and seemed as polished and precise as the sophisticated equipment in her laboratories.

Dr. Przedpelska chaired the Department of Neurophysiology of Movement at the Institute of Orthopaedics and Rehabilitation Medicine in Poznan. Her empire consisted of six rooms at the institute, each filled with sensitive electronic equipment used to identify, evaluate, and quantify neurological disorders.

Poznan is a factory town. Its workers spend their days wrestling with heavy machinery that vibrates with power and energy. As a result, the institute has seen a continual stream of men and women complaining of numbness or tingling in their hands and other problems similar to and including carpal tunnel syndrome. This was my introduction to the difficulties of clinical research — research conducted on human beings. People in general are a complicated and not always cooperative lot, possessed of a host of hidden variables. But working with human beings was always rewarding, if for no other reason than when research finds benefits, they can go into immediate application.

Dr. Przedpelska's daughter, Elzbieta, and I worked three afternoons a week in the laboratories, carrying out neurosensory testing on men and women who had what then was called "vibratory disease." We used some complicated and advanced technology to evaluate the performance of neural networks. The goal was to design exercises and interventions that would improve their health without involving surgery.

It was important work. The men who came in had callused hands and arms and muscles that bulged even when they picked up a cup of coffee. They smelled of cheap soap, sweat, and strong tobacco, and though they often joked about the web of wires and sensors we attached, we could feel their underlying sense of concern. If they couldn't feel anything in their hands, they couldn't work the equipment. If they couldn't work the equipment, they wouldn't have a job.

The experience of translating research into clinical benefits for patients I'd treated as a young third-year medical student has remained with me throughout my career. I now see that research is as essential to patient care as aspirin, antibiotics, and scalpels.

WHEN I ENTERED medical school in Poznan in the early 1970s, the women's rights movement was sweeping the United States. I didn't notice. I'd started on a career training path that was at least 12 years long and uphill most of the way. My fellow students and I had no time to pay attention to the details of a women's revolution in a country so far away. Readers in the United States, especially those for whom the women's rights movement is part of their history, might be surprised to learn that in Poland the medical profession was already dominated by women.

In the United States, sexual bias created the imbalance in the roles men and women occupied in society, and reaction to that bias changed those roles. In Poland, World War II tipped the balance. One of civilization's darkest eras consumed 5.6 million Poles, 16 percent of the nation's population. Most of those lost were men in their prime.

As a result, women were encouraged to take jobs and pursue careers that under other circumstances would have been the sole province of men. I remember going with friends to the movies in which the feature attraction was preceded by shorts depicting healthy, tanned women smiling and waving as they piloted tractors through fields of yellow grain. These films were a little strange; it was hard to believe anyone would enjoy driving a tractor as much as these women.

The gender imbalance was such that men were given inducements in the form of extra points on entrance exams if they chose to pursue careers in certain professions, including medicine. However, both men and women were usually drawn to other professions because the paychecks came sooner. A great range of degrees could be acquired in four to six years, but young people entering medical school faced six years of formal education followed by six or more years of residency training before they became independent practitioners.

Once certified, physicians just beginning their careers earned little more than they had as residents. In fact, there was little difference in salaries among all professions. Wages were set by the government. As a result young Poles who chose careers in medicine did so for no other reason than their desire to be doctors. This may not have attracted the most ambitious people in our society, but it certainly drew the most dedicated and conscientious.

When I look back over my career I find it hard to identify many instances when I was affected by gender discrimination. In the United States, I did encounter some prejudice, but it was directed more toward my national background. There were a few times in orthopedics when my gender raised a few eyebrows.

MEDICINE IS WORK. I'm not talking about long hours spent reading medical texts under bad lighting or 20-hour days and seven-day weeks, though there's plenty of that. I'm talking about sheer physical labor, the kind that makes you sweat and leaves your muscles aching to the point of immobility. Orthopedics, the first specialty I entered, is particularly demanding of young residents. Orthopedics comprises treatments and procedures that repair or restore skeletal structures and the tissues that support them. Every structure, from the smallest bones in a child's finger to the massive hips of professional wrestlers, falls within the province of the orthopedist.

Orthopedic procedures directed at bones and joints can be long and tedious. Residents learn these procedures by assisting in surgery, often by standing at the surgeon's side and applying just the right amount of force to the patient's leg or arm so that the structure the surgeon is working on remains open and accessible. Most young residents are surprised by the amount of force needed to hold a leg stable while a surgeon works on a hip. The delicacy of movement needed to situate the joint or limb in the right position and the need for absolute stability are other aspects of procedures that assisting residents must get used to. Not only is a certain degree of force required to rotate a pelvis or leg, but it must also be done correctly and gently.

Even hand surgery can be arduous. A resident's job in these procedures is to pull gently on the hooks and surgical attachments that draw tissue away from the bony structures the surgeon is working on. Imagine looping a small rubber band around the handle of a full coffee cup resting on a table. Pick up a pair of tweezers and pull on the rubber band so that it stretches away from the cup but does not move it. Now hold it that way for an hour and a half. You can change hands every so often, but the rubber band has to remain stretched and the liquid in the cup should show no ripples.

I'm not a large woman. I stand five feet five inches and weigh about 122 pounds. I have no doubt that during my residencies and my studies as a fellow, a surgeon or two may have been a little concerned about my physical abilities when I scrubbed in for a major hip operation or similar procedure. But I did what needed to be done. What I lacked in muscle I made up for in determination. The perseverance and patience I learned while pulling steadily on a leg or section of tissue during a hip replacement would serve me well in unanticipated circumstances such as arguing the possibility and potential of a face transplant before the institutional review board of one of the world's leading medical institutions.

One of the more important lessons residents learn by standing beside an experienced surgeon under the bright lights of an operating room (OR) is how to give clear, concise instructions. Medical literature often describes a surgeon as conducting a procedure. Working with experienced associates, residents, and nurses is often like leading an orchestra through a symphony. Every player knows what's expected, what to do, and when to do it. All it takes for a cellist to move from forte to fortissimo is a nod from the conductor. All it takes for a resident to put a little more tension on a joint is a single word from a surgeon. It works regardless of the gender of those involved. During routine procedures, residents and nurses know by heart the sequence of events, the instruments and materials that will be needed. It's not unusual for surgeons working with experienced teams to find a pair of forceps or other surgical instrument being placed in their outstretched hands before they have a chance to ask for it.

The challenge of surgery comes when the surgeon ventures into the unknown, such as when revising an earlier procedure or removing a cancer. Medicine has a host of truly remarkable imaging technologies such as X-rays, magnetic resonance imaging (MRI), and computed tomography (CT), but surgeons never know what an organ is going to look like until they see it. Just as you cannot really diagnose an illness in a patient by looking at a photograph, you cannot really understand the nature of a trauma by looking at an MRI. The flesh must be laid bare before you.

Challenging procedures require extensive preparation. X-rays, MRIs, CT scans, and other images are reviewed again and again. The procedure and all its details will be conducted in the surgeon's imagination again and again. And still there will be surprises. Novel and complicated procedures are conducted with great deliberation. Proceeding slowly is an impossible luxury because almost all operations are conducted with a clock running. The challenge of doing them right belongs to the surgeon. The labor falls on the residents.

Forgive me if I've created the impression that there was no discrimination in Polish medical schools. There was, but it was between generations rather than genders — between older, experienced doctors who held authority and determined policy, and younger, energetic residents determined to make the world, or at least the department, better.

A young male colleague and I were given the responsibility of directing the efforts of the journal club. Each of us would select two papers or studies from the medical literature for discussion among ourselves, other residents, and the senior members of the department. This wasn't a book club or a literary discussion group. Discussion of papers advancing new ideas for surgical procedures and new concepts of tissue functions, often at cellular or even molecular levels, required forethought and preparation. The discussions were pleasant and focused, and they advanced our medical knowledge of the field. However, my colleague and I felt the advances were not moving either far enough or fast enough. We began to push for more work. We advocated that the residents present three papers and that an additional three be presented by the senior staff.

The senior staff didn't exactly greet our proposal with enthusiasm. They folded their arms across their chests and settled more deeply into the depressions they had worn into their chairs over the years.

Anyone who is young and ambitious knows what it's like to present a new idea to a senior official only to be greeted with silence, a raised eyebrow, and an expression that says, *Look, kid, we've been doing it this way ever since I can remember. The system works. It's comfortable, and I'm comfortable in it. Don't make waves.*

We paid no attention to these expressions of cool disapproval. We relentlessly drove to expand the number of journals being reviewed.

There came a day when one of the senior doctors called us aside and said simply, "Don't push."

You remember the tone in your father's voice when you were ten and he turned to you and quietly said, "Don't."

You knew he wasn't speaking out of exasperation or willful authority. He just said "don't," and you knew deep in your gut that you'd better not. That was the tone in the senior doctor's voice, and of course we listened. I still hear that tone now and again at symposia and medical society meetings when a young resident or fellow pushes a new idea too forcefully.

Our idea of reviewing more journals was a good one. If the head of a department or a senior doctor had advanced the proposal, the response would have been "Why didn't we think of that earlier?"

So I learned to evaluate an idea first, to determine its worth on its merits, and only then to consider its origins. I've also found that the more ideas I listen to, the more good ideas I'm offered. There's nothing warmer than the light in a young fellow's eyes when you tell him, "You might be onto something there. That's worth exploring."

There was an advantage to being a female resident in orthopedics in a Polish medical school in the 1970s: I had company. Dr. Tomaszewska chaired the department of rehabilitative medicine. The vice-chair and the chiefs of all the divisions were also women. This proved to be something of a comfort during 1977.

That winter was like all Polish winters. The days were cold and short, the nights long and dark, and every wind that blew was filled with snow. We spent that winter doing what we have always done in winter. We danced.

We drove away the cold and dark with music, balls, dances, festivals, and parties of all sorts. *Karnawal*, "carnival" in Polish, stretched across the emptiest part of the year from the end of Christmas holidays until Ash Wednesday in Lent and filled the span with color, sound, and motion. It was during one of the carnival dances with lights ablaze and music filling the hall that my stomach started dancing with me.

At first I thought it might have been something I'd eaten. But the nausea persisted. I was like all women: pregnancy is the first thing you suspect and the last thing you believe. Our son Krzysztof — Kris — was born nine months after the ball was over.

During the 1970s in Poland, there were few institutions or businesses that didn't grant a woman at least six weeks of maternity leave. My husband, Wlodzimierz (Vlodek for short), and I shared the responsibility of raising young Kris. Just as I was often on call at the clinic, we were both on call when it came to Kris. And I must admit that there were times when he was far more demanding than any department chairman.

Kris's birth led me to the first and only overt instance of gender discrimination that I can remember. I wanted desperately to be a hand surgeon and applied for a residency in the orthopedic department's hand-surgery clinic. There was only one opening and there were many candidates who wanted to fill it. The chair of the department knew me and knew of my interest in hand surgery and was familiar with my research in neurophysiology and nerve regeneration.

All this qualified me for the position, but there was one indiscreet question that needed to be answered and the chairman asked it without hesitation: was I planning on having more children?

Today this question would land both the chairman and the institution in a pot of legal trouble, but I understood it completely. Hand surgery was a very limited specialty. Few others could perform the procedures, so hand surgeons were on call almost all the time. If a surgeon was unable to get to the clinic at a moment's notice, a young man or woman would be at increased risk of losing the use of a hand or limb, or of losing the appendage completely.

I told the chairman that I was happy with the family I had and that I had no intention of expanding it. I was soon chosen as an assistant professor, becoming the youngest member of the department. I left a world where most of my colleagues were women and entered a realm where nearly all would be men. There were 25 faculty members at the institution, of which only three were women, including me.

I worked. Vlodek worked. Kris grew. Life was full, busy, and normal for four years.

CHAPTER 5

Becoming a Microsurgeon

IT WAS A SATURDAY in Finland, early 1980, with winter still heavy on the land. At that latitude, the days are short and time reckoned by sunrise or sunset can be confusing, but I remember that it was afternoon. The young man arrived at the hospital on a gurney. His hand came in on ice in a box.

He and his friends had been chopping firewood. His hand had been at the wrong place at the wrong time. The details of the accident didn't matter, although no doubt they remain forever seared into the young woodchopper's memory: the thud of the ax, the crunch of bone, and the sudden realization that the object looking so out of place on the ground next to his muddy boot was his hand.

His life changed on that gray day.

So did mine.

I'd come to what was then called the Orthopaedic Hospital of the Invalid Foundation (it is now ORTON Orthopaedic Hospital) in Helsinki to study with the noted Finnish microsurgeon Dr. Simo Vilkki. It had been a two-day trip on a passenger ferry from Poland's northern port of Gdansk to Helsinki on the southern coast of Finland. During the day, my fellow travelers and I would look over the railings to see icebergs moving lazily through the dark Baltic Sea. At night, we lay in our berths, listening to the throbbing engines and the cold waves beating against the hull, and wondered where the icebergs were.

I arrived in March at the great port city to begin two months of training in hand surgery. Owing to the complexity of the anatomy involved, this is a particularly challenging specialty. Hold your hand to your face and wriggle your thumb and fingers. There are 27 bones controlled by 28 muscles. Your hand can grasp a baseball bat and pick up a needle; it's strong enough to crush an orange and sensitive enough to pick up a feather without disturbing its shape; it knows hot and cold and pain. When the nerves, tendons, veins, and arteries that serve this wonderfully engineered mechanism are severed, say by a misdirected ax, it takes hour upon long hour to reconnect everything and restore some degree of utility.

I suspect that it was because hand surgeries are exceedingly long endeavors that Dr. Vilkki called me. After all, it was a Saturday and the hospital's residents, some with greater experience than mine, were all conveniently indisposed. None seemed to want to spend the afternoon, night, and most of Sunday morning in an operating room. But I saw the opportunity to scrub in with Dr. Vilkki as a gift, an unexpected bit of fortune borne of misfortune. At the risk of sounding callous, I can testify that amputations are rare events and the opportunity to watch and assist one of the Europe's most skilled surgeons, a pioneer in hand surgery, was an opportunity indeed.

The hand had been severed just above the wrist. The patient was lucky. If the ax had fallen below the wrist, it could have wrecked some very delicate and complex anatomical structures. He was also fortunate that the instrument had been an ax. Many lose limbs in horrible automobile or industrial accidents that leave the limbs too mangled to reconstruct and reattach.

The woodchopper's hand, pale and lifeless, was not in terrible shape, but it needed debridement (the cleaning and removal of contaminated tissue). Arteries and veins had to be cleaned of dirt, debris, and clotted blood.

Nerves, ligaments, and tendons had to be identified and prepared for reattachment to their counterparts on the patient's arm.

Dr. Vilkki and I were in one room cleaning the delicate structures of the hand. Other doctors were in an adjacent room preparing the end of the man's arm. There are tricks that surgeons use to identify small anatomical structures. We mark a vein by slipping a suture (surgical thread) though it and snipping both ends of the thread short. Longer sutures mark arteries. Nerves may be identified by a suture with one long end and one short end. When the hand and arm are debrided and juxtaposed with the marked nerves, arteries, veins, and tendons, it soon becomes apparent which structures are to be attached to one another.

For several hours Dr. Vilkki and I bent over the hand. We spoke quietly to each other, noting the appearance of an artery, the location of a nerve, the damage to a tendon, but for the most part we worked in silence, focusing on the pale object before us. When we finished, the hand was wrapped in a towel and carried into the operating room on a tray.

The appendage was lifeless and had been kept cold intentionally. Chilling almost any tissue extends its viability by slowing cellular metabolism. One of the things aspiring surgeons must get used to after working in the warmth of a patient's body and blood is picking up a chilled organ or extremity. The anesthetized patient's arm lay on a table beside him. The hand and arm were brought together and the reattachment procedure began. Bones are joined first to give stability to the arm and hand, and to allow the remainder of the work to proceed. There were the sounds that attend operating rooms the world over: the small whirr, tick, and beep of various electronic monitors and machines, the soft wheeze of ventilators, the clatter of instruments being dropped into trays.

Scalpels and clamps fall with a jangle. Microsurgical needles barely make a sound. The average human hair is 60 to 90 microns (a micron is one millionth of a meter) thick, whereas microsurgical needles range in diameter from 40 microns to 100 microns. It would require a microscope to thread them, so they come with sutures attached. After several sutures are placed, the thread becomes too short to use. The needle is discarded, dropped into a tray with a tick; the surgeon takes another, stretches his or her neck, perhaps flexes a hand, and bends back over the work and into a world of minute veins, arteries, nerves, and tendons circumscribed by the view through the microscope's lens.

There was a very distinct moment in the procedure

that remains with me today. When the arteries and veins were connected, Dr. Vilkki spoke quietly to a nurse. She released a clamp and blood began to flow. The color of the hand went from pale to pink. As it turned from a lifeless assembly of shattered bones and flesh destined for a surgical waste bin into a structure that once again might hold a cup of coffee or wipe a tear from a child's face, I knew immediately what my medical specialty would be: I was going to be a hand surgeon.

My amazement at the rejuvenation of the hand was easily exceeded by the expression on the patient's face when he came out of the fog of anesthesia. He had gone to sleep knowing that his hand had been chopped off, and he awoke to find it reattached. His expression of wonder and gratitude only reinforced the decision I had made as the hand began to turn pink.

This remarkable transplant is more accurately described as an autograft or hand "replant" since the patient's own limb was reattached. A true transplant, or allograft, involves transplanting limbs, tissues, or organs from one individual to another. In the majority of instances, this would involve material from a donor who is deceased, but this is not the case in all instances, such as a kidney transplant. On many occasions, the technical or surgical challenge is greater with a replant than with a transplant — a donated hand will not have suffered the trauma or damage seen in one severed by an ax or a piece of farm machinery. Yet the greatest difference between an autograft and allograft is that the latter requires that the patient make a lifelong commitment to a strict regimen of taking drugs to suppress the immune system's rejection of the foreign limb. This is no small consideration and is the primary reason why candidates for transplant procedures undergo intensive psychological screening. The world's first hand transplant is illustrative of the problem and challenge facing patients.

ON SEPTEMBER 25, 1998, at the Edouard Herriot Hospital in Lyon, France, Dr. Jean-Michel Dubernard joined Dr. Earl Owen of Sydney, Australia, Dr. Nadey Hakim of London, England, and an international team of surgeons to transplant the hand of a recently deceased motorcyclist to the arm of forty-eight-year-old Clint Hallam, who had flown to France from his home in Perth, Australia, for the procedure. The operation took 14 hours and was considered a major triumph. The triumph crumbled three years later when Mr. Hallam arrived at St. Mary's Hospital, London. There Dr. Hakim spent 90 minutes amputating the hand that he and other surgeons had labored over for hours in France.

"I hold myself responsible for a good part in that I allowed this to happen," Mr. Hallam told *The New York Times* shortly after the hand had been removed. "I am fully responsible for the rejection of this hand, which was satisfactory before I stopped my drugs."

Hallam explained that he had begun the enterprise with the best of intentions but had gradually lost his determination to follow the regimen of exercise and drugs. His doctors reported that he failed to appear for scheduled checkups and that blood tests showed that his compliance with the drug regimen had been intermittent. Although the transplantation of a new hand to Mr. Hallam's arm was by all parameters a technical success, most surgeons would regard the overall operation as a failure. Such a loss can be doubly frustrating because there is little that a doctor can do when a patient gives up.

Dr. Dubernard achieved another first in 2005 when he and another team successfully completed a partial face transplant from a cadaver to 38-year-old Isabelle Dinoire, whose face had been mauled by a dog. Ms. Dinoire made her treating physicians more than a little nervous when she lit a cigarette and returned to her smoking habit several weeks after the surgery. Smoking can exert a powerful effect on the immune system and is to be discouraged in any transplant patient receiving a hand, face, kidney, liver, or any other organ or structure. She is now doing well, and is integrated back into her community.

Stories such as this highlight one of the major challenges facing any surgeon or physician contemplating a procedure that had never before been performed on a human being. A patient's physiology can easily be described. The patient's psyche is far more intangible and slippery.

AFTER THE HAND replantation surgery, I let it be known that I'd be happy to return if the Invalid Foundation would invite me. A little over 12 months later, in July 1981, I was again on the ferry churning north through the dark Baltic Sea to Helsinki. This time, the waves were tipped with pearl-white foam and bright glints of sunshine instead of ice.

The Helsinki I found in the summer was not the Helsinki I had known in the winter. I was limited to a budget of about $200 a month, a sum that did not go far even when stretched as thin as possible. I lived and ate at the hospital and spent the weekend pedaling around the city's museums, gardens, and shops on a rented bicycle. Bus fare, though reasonable, was not in a young surgical fellow's budget. I spent my days with colleagues, learning as much as I could about surgical technique. I spent the nights with rats in the hospital basement.

Animals have always been essential to medical progress. Science has yet to develop a model or substance that in any way replicates the look and feel of living tissue. To learn to join the separate ends of a nerve, to learn to quickly and efficiently reconnect a severed artery, you must work in vivo: you must work in life with real tissue and a clock running. Cells need the oxygen supplied by blood coursing through arteries. They can survive without it for a limited time. When that limit is reached, the cells begin to perish and no surgeon, however skilled, has the ability to restore life to them. The clock starts running when the artery is severed. For a surgeon restoring or replacing a limb or organ, concentration and patience are virtues that must be supplemented with certainty, speed, and skill.

The skills to be applied in the operating rooms on the upper floors of the hospital were sharpened in the institution's laboratory. After a day in the OR or in wards caring for patients, I'd go to the basement microsurgery lab that lay at the end of a long, silent, and shadowy corridor.

The small room was furnished with an operating table, a large microsurgery microscope, and walls of shelves holding test tubes, jars, dishes, and scientific glassware of all types that reflected the room's lights in small, dull glints.

The surgical microscope was reasonably modern compared to the one I had used at medical school in Poznan. Such a microsurgical microscope bears little resemblance to the microscopes you may remember from movies and high school laboratories. The modern microsurgical microscopes are bifocal instruments that stand as tall as a surgeon or even taller. They are suspended from cantilevers attached to heavy pedestals that give them stability while procedures are being conducted. Most modern microsurgical microscopes have foot controls to allow the surgeon to adjust the instrument's focus while keeping his or her hands involved in the work beneath the lens. Some of the more advanced instruments in use today can be controlled by voice command. The surgeon's hands never have to leave the work.

The room where the animals were kept, the vivarium, was adjacent to the lab. An animal would be taken from its cage and weighed on a small scale in the lab. The animal's weight determined the amount of anesthetic that would be required to keep it immobile and free of pain. It would be prepped and laid on the operating bed. Instruments would be arranged on a tray. The scope would be moved into place and the procedure would begin. With my eyes pressed against the microscope, instruments in hand, and my mind on the magnified anatomy beneath me, I felt the room grow so still that it seemed removed not only from the hospital, but also the world. The hours would pass silently, like leaves falling from a tree.

When the evening's work was complete, the animal would be returned to its cage to recover, the instruments sterilized, the room cleaned, the lights turned off, and the door locked. I'd retrace my steps along the shadowy corridors to the hospital's dormitory, where I was living while in Helsinki. The next day seemed to begin the moment my head hit the pillow.

HUMANITY OWES A substantial debt to the rat. Rats in laboratories provide the opportunity to discover how different living tissues respond to drugs. They are also the stage on which microsurgeons hone existing skills and develop new ones. Twenty years ago, I spent evenings in the hospital basement, reconnecting animal limbs using my newly acquired microsurgical techniques. The experience I gathered during those long, solitary nights peering through magnifying lenses while sliding a needle through the thin vessels and nerves of an anesthetized animal have benefited countless patients. Many years later, when it became obvious that a face transplant was feasible, we once again turned to the rat to study how such a procedure might be performed and to prove that it could be safely accomplished.

The work that I was doing in the hospital's laboratory was more than mere practice. It contributed critical data and observations to an ongoing study of surgical techniques. Surgeons have no secrets — rather, they keep no secrets. If they find or develop a tool or technique that confers the slightest advantage over existing tools and techniques, the first thing they do is to tell everybody about it in exhaustive detail in published papers and at medical symposia. My work with animals in the hospital basement was distilled into a carefully worded study to be presented at the Scandinavian Society for Surgery of the Hand, held that year in the university city of Örebro, Sweden. Because of my work and contributions derived from long hours in the quiet basement, Dr. Kauko Solonen, chairman of the Invalid Foundation's Hand Surgery Department, invited me to tag along to the meeting.

Medical meetings are curious gatherings — a mixture of science, socializing, and business. In the carpeted halls of convention centers or grand hotels, surgeons known around the world for their skill and accomplishments grab one another's hands, laugh, tell jokes (usually bad ones), and behave in general as if they were uncles, aunts, and second cousins gathering for a family reunion.

The doctors are frequently accosted by beaming representatives of drug companies and manufacturers of medical devices, who invite them to try out this new scalpel or that new microscope, hear the merits of this new drug, and get a free coffee cup or bag of golf balls emblazoned with the company's logo. When the time comes, everyone files into an auditorium, where they listen with remarkable patience to introductory remarks from someone who has the tedious responsibility of thanking everyone remotely associated with creating the symposium.

The hall then grows dark and quiet as a slide projector casts a PowerPoint image of a section of anatomy on a large screen beside the shadowy podium. The larger symposia may have half a dozen of these screens around the room, broadcasting the presentation via closed-circuit television to select rooms throughout the convention center and perhaps to a few rooms in centers or hospitals on the other side of the world. One by one, some of the best hand surgeons in the world walk to the podium to describe how they approached this problem or resolved that one. Their display of skill, their knowledge of anatomy, and the certainty with which they described their procedures and techniques left me all the more certain after the conference in Sweden that I would pursue a career in microsurgery.

THE FIRST THING I did upon returning home to Poznan was to introduce my colleagues to the microsurgical techniques I had learned in Finland. We worked with pigs' feet acquired from local butchers (who no doubt wondered about the curious culinary tastes the doctors at their local hospital seemed to have developed). I was able to show my colleagues what I had learned in the Helsinki hospital basement about applying microsurgical techniques to minute arteries and veins. The directors of the institution saw the worth of this training and came up with a small budget that allowed us to acquire a used operating microscope that would enable us to place sutures into structures barely visible to the naked eye.

It was 1985 when Dr. Vilkki, who by this time had become a friend, contacted me. I was serving my last year as chief resident in hand surgery at the Institute for Orthopaedics and Rehabilitation Medicine at the Karol Marcinkowski University of Medical Sciences in Poznan. Dr. Vilkki informed me of a weeklong series of courses on hand surgery to be offered in Ljubljana, Yugoslavia (now Slovenia). They would be taught by a number of remarkable doctors, including a renowned team from a private hand-surgery clinic associated with the Department of Orthopaedic Surgery at the School of Medicine at the University of Louisville in Louisville, Kentucky.

The surgeons in Louisville are considered to be among the best in the world. Dr. Vilkki had been to Louisville and knew the institute's surgeons well. He advised me to write to Dr. Harold Kleinert, who had founded the University of Louisville Hand Clinic in 1953 and made it one of the foremost in the world (it is now Kleinert, Kutz, and Associates Hand Care Center). I was to ask to be considered for a fellowship in his department. Dr. Vilkki had already written Dr. Kleinert and told him of my assistance in the Finnish hand replantation and of my work in Poznan.

This was too much to believe. This was Louisville! The small clinic and hospital in the middle of horse country was home to some of the best microsurgeons in the world and had a commensurate reputation. To say, "I'm going to Louisville for a fellowship" is equivalent to a ballplayer saying, "I'm going to the New York Yankees' training camp."

But there were obstacles. Even if I were invited, I didn't have the money for a plane ticket to go to Louisville to interview for the fellowship. Even if I could find it, I didn't have the bureaucratic qualifications or contacts that would allow me to acquire a visa as a medical trainee. Poznan, Poland, was on the wrong side of the Iron Curtain. The possibility of studying at the Kentucky clinic seemed to be fading faster than it had arisen.

This problem had a solution. Dr. Vilkki told me that Dr. Graham Lister, director of residency programs in Louisville, would be attending the Ljubljana symposium to present courses and lectures. He noted that while in Europe, Dr. Lister would also be conducting interviews to identify potential candidates for fellowships.

I had to get to Ljubljana. The organizer of the Ljubljana educational symposium was Dr. Marco Godina, then a busy young microsurgeon with a growing reputation. (The American Society for Reconstructive Microsurgery now offers an annual fellowship in his honor.) Dr. Godina made some calls and arranged for me to stay in a student dormitory on the campus of Ljubljana University. He was also able to get the fee for the microsurgery course waived.

Airfare was beyond consideration, so for three very long days I rode in a passenger coach as the train rattled south from Poznan in west central Poland though what was then Czechoslovakia and Hungary to Ljubljana, which lies just north of the Adriatic Sea. The distance between Poznan and Ljubljana is about 500 or more miles as the crow flies, and considerably farther if the crow follows the railroad tracks that weave and twist through valleys, hills, and the eastern reaches of the Alps. About the second day of the trip, the charm of the passing hills and villages began to wear off.

I arrived at the university tired, shaken, but ready to learn. Dr. Lister had brought a coterie of Louisville surgical fellows with him to help with instruction. Immediately I began to pester them with questions about what he was like, what sorts of questions he might ask during the interviews, what was he looking for in a potential fellow. Most responded to these questions with a smile and a polite "Don't worry." They had obviously heard many of these questions before. There was a swarm of European surgeons in attendance for the course and interviews. This was, after all, Louisville, an institution where a young fellow would get training from some of the best microsurgeons in the world and would scrub in on dozens of cases of amputations and the replantation of hands, fingers, toes, and other limbs.

One of the American fellows gave me invaluable advice.

"Remember — with Lister, be forthright," he said. "Don't exaggerate. Don't make things up."

During the interview, the doctor complimented my command of English and asked many of the questions I had anticipated. Why was I interested in hand surgery? Why did I want to come to the United States? What were my goals? He then asked me some very specific questions about the anatomy of the hand. I hesitated for only a moment, remembered the advice, and told him I could not answer.

He asked why.

I explained that my colleagues and I had only limited access to cadavers, a problem that severely handicapped our education.

He nodded. I think he understood that the eager young candidate before him was just being honest.

I consider two qualities inherent in my character responsible for whatever success I may have achieved in medicine: I always want to learn, and I am forthright.

Soon after the interview, Dr. Lister told me that I had won the fellowship and would be able to start my training within three years.

The three-day ride back to Poznan seemed to take only minutes. The villages and hills flew by. I didn't care. I was going to Louisville, or as I learned to say, "Loo'v'l."

Looking back on those days, back to all the operations and books and nights in the basement with rats, and then to the interview with Dr. Lister, I find a certain irony in thinking that it was not what I knew, but what

I had told the doctor I didn't know that put me on this long, circuitous path to the United States, where I would one day lean over to look at a patient about to receive a new face.

CHAPTER 6

The Face Is Different from the Heart

WHEN THE TRAIN that carried me from the microsurgery conference and interview with Dr. Lister arrived in Poznan, the fellowship in Louisville lay three years ahead. First, I had to complete my doctorate. These were difficult years for my country. In August 1980, some 17,000 workers seized the Lenin Shipyard in Gdansk, Poland, to protest working and living conditions. The government, which normally would have responded with immediate force, instead hesitated, then stepped back. Mieczyslaw Jagielski, Poland's prime minister, signed an agreement with Lech Walesa, leader of the strikers. The pact granted the workers the right to organize and strike. The effect on the general populace was electric. Hope for reform and a degree of independence blossomed and thrived for 18 months.

But on December 13, 1981, Poles awoke to find their country under martial law. The borders were closed, airports were shut down, and travel between cities required a permit. A curfew was imposed from 10 p.m. to 6 a.m., and the streets of Poland's great cities and small towns sank into a cold, dark silence. The military took control of nearly every aspect of the economy, from public administration to health services to the nation's mines, ports, and railway stations. Thousands were arrested overnight. Thousands more were questioned. A chill settled on the nation. It would remain for two years until martial law was lifted.

Kris was four years old and totally unaware of the grim political situation, or so I thought. But the art he began to bring home from school was devoid of color. Everything — people, cars, animals — was drawn in black crayon on white paper. When martial law was lifted in the summer of 1983, color returned to the land and to Kris's drawings. To this day I have no idea why my child's kindergarten artwork seemed to have absorbed the mood of the nation.

For me, those trying times were filled with work, work, and more work.

I spent my days caring for patients in the orthopedics ward and my nights and weekends placing sutures in the veins of rabbits in the university's microsurgery lab. Work in the lab seemed endless. The research was part of my doctoral thesis, which had to be completed and presented not once but several times before I could shove my clothes into a suitcase and board the plane for the United States.

The procedure for developing a doctoral thesis in Poland is part tradition, part education, part science, and part politics. The parts are not equal.

The long march to acquiring a doctorate begins with selecting a mentor, someone who will serve as a teacher, guide, and taskmaster. A mentor also serves as protector, deflecting the slings and arrows launched by other students and officials within the academy.

Some of the arrows are pure scientific criticism and are valuable. Some of the barbs are political. Rivalries and jealousies abound within universities, and one professor may take the opportunity to settle a score with another by taking a few pokes at the latter's young thesis candidate. There is little that a mentor can do to deflect these criticisms and even less that a candidate can do to dodge them. But a good mentor can and should take appropriate note of politically inflicted wounds by offering such comforting words as "Oh, just ignore Professor So-and-So. He's still upset because I won a grant 12 years ago, and he didn't. I also dated his wife before they were married. Get on with the work."

Sometimes students seek out mentors, and sometimes mentors choose the students. A student who can find a mentor respected in a specific field may get a significant head start on a path to a promising career in that field. Not only is a young PhD recognized for having studied under a well-known master, but the mentor can also bring real influence to bear when it comes to recommending the protégé to institutions or providing an introduction to the chairman of an important department. On the other hand, a promising student will be sought out by a professor with an eye to a future time when the student's work will reflect favorably on the teacher. Yet, it's not always about politics. In most instances, in order to learn as much as possible, a student seeks a mentor who is an instructor in the student's chosen area of study.

My mentor, Professor Alfons Senger, MD, chairman of Poznan's department of orthopedics, was a tall, slim, strongly built man who had a full head of black hair well into his 60s. His dark eyes glinted beneath a perpetually furrowed brow. Although his demeanor was often stern, it was never off-putting or discouraging. I always thought that if he weren't a highly respected surgeon, he'd have been a famous general, one of those somber men depicted in larger-than-life oil portraits, one hand on a sword and the other resting on a map, seemingly indifferent to the battle raging in the background.

The doctor and I created a thesis and designed the experiments that would test and (we hoped) advance the thesis. Together we presented the proposal to the orthopedics faculty. After I answered a few questions, I was asked to step outside into the long hall with its high arched ceilings. Eventually, Dr. Senger stepped into the hall to inform me that the orthopedics faculty had approved the thesis and he was now required to present the idea to the medical school senate.

The senate, a body of some 200 physician professors, convenes on one Wednesday every month. It has been doing so since the institution was founded and continues the practice to this day. The men and women of the senate gather in the great hall to discuss promotions, business, and school issues as well as to whisper the latest gossip. At some point during the meeting, a physician-mentor will present the outline of a thesis being proposed by one of his students. The faculty will consider it, ask a few questions, and vote. A simple majority carries the day.

Following one of these meetings, Dr. Senger emerged

from the hall to tell me that I would have three years to complete a dissertation entitled *The Evaluation of Different Microsurgical Techniques of Arterial Anastomosis in the Diameter Below One Millimeter: An Experimental Study in Rabbits.* I'd also have to publish at least 21 articles on this subject or related ones in peer-reviewed journals, and I was expected to present interim studies and abstracts at varied medical symposia and meetings around Europe. Louisville suddenly seemed to be a thousand years away and getting farther away by the minute.

The lab that was to occupy so many evenings over the next three years was in the Institute of Orthopaedics and Rehabilitation at 26 Czerwca Street. The building was once part of a cluster of structures housing an order of Carmelite nuns. At some point in its long history it had been converted to clinical use, but the transformation was never completed. The building was filled with long halls, high ceilings, arched stained-glass windows, deep shadows, and the ghosts of silent women hurrying to vespers with their heads bowed.

The microsurgery lab was on the third floor in the department of hand surgery, at the end of a long hall in which the heavy doors of doctors' offices stood like silent sentinels. It wasn't the sort of lab that comes readily to mind and probably fits better into a bad Hollywood movie about mad scientists than a place where surgical skills are explored and perfected. A fixture in the high arched ceiling cast an unflattering light onto the autoclave, the table where the animals were prepared, the scale where they were weighed to determine the anesthesia they should receive, and the microsurgical microscope.

The instrument that looked so out of place in the old Carmelite convent was far from modern. To adjust it, the surgeon had to set his or her instruments down and grasp different knobs to adjust the magnification or move the viewing field. With a little practice one could do this without glancing up from the eyepiece. It was an awkward instrument by today's standards but sufficient for young doctors polishing their microsurgical skills or completing a thesis on innovative ways to place sutures in minuscule arteries and veins.

Once a procedure starts, whether on animal or man, it cannot be interrupted until it is completed. A severed artery or vein means a region of the body is being deprived of blood and that the cells in that region are beginning to slide toward death. At a certain point, the slide becomes irreversible. The period between the interruption of blood flow and irreversible tissue death is known as the ischemic time, and it varies from organ to organ and tissue to tissue. Every surgeon knows these times. One of the great challenges of surgery is to complete a procedure and restore blood flow before this crucial point in time passes.

In mammals — human beings as well as rabbits — the popliteal artery is the primary artery delivering blood to the lower leg. It's a sizable artery in people, but in a rabbit, it's small, about the size of the lead in a mechanical pencil.

The thrust of my thesis was to create and evaluate techniques for the joining of two vessels, anastomosis, that were efficient, reliable, effective, and durable. This involved anesthetizing the rabbit, severing the artery, and rejoining its ends with different suturing techniques and materials. Then I'd allow the rabbit to heal and examine the restored vein microscopically to learn how the animal's self-restorative systems had reacted to the procedure. Often, a vein or artery will look beautiful on the outside, but a closer look at the lumen — the interior of the artery — will show it to be scarred, clogged with thrombi (clots), or significantly reduced in diameter. All these characteristics are problematic because they limit or even cut off blood flow to the legs, leading to necrosis (cell death) and no other clinical choice but to amputate.

A blood vessel is composed of layers of cells, creating tubes within tubes. Each layer has specific functions and each can influence the actions of the others. If two ends of a vein or artery are poorly joined, circulating blood cells may snag on the juncture. Other cells adhere to these, and gradually or rapidly a clot will grow that will either diminish blood flow, block the artery entirely, or break free to meander through the circulatory system and lodge elsewhere in the body with dire consequences.

All the aspects and outcomes of the anastomotic procedures I was exploring had to be documented in exacting detail, often photographed, and then interpreted. It wasn't enough to note how the various suture patterns affected the artery's patency (the degree to which it was open or unobstructed) and healing. It was necessary to understand and explain why one suture pattern created a wound that healed over a certain period of time and looked a certain way compared to the results produced by another suture pattern. Cells were stained and examined for minute changes in their interiors that might be related to the sutures.

At the end of a long night, the lab was cleaned and the instruments were sterilized. The animals would be gently carried down three flights of steps, through halls that linked the institution's other buildings, and into the vivarium where they were kept and cared for.

Once a month, I'd submit observations and results to Dr. Senger. After a few days the paper came back, sometimes with more red ink scribbled on it than there was of my original black ink. Questions would be answered and corrections made. More experiments would be conducted, again the results would be presented, and again the paper would reappear days later, drenched in red.

As the months passed and the clinical results began to show a definite direction, the red ink began to disappear. The paper began to take shape. Finally I had a stack of nearly 200 typed pages and photographs that constituted the final draft of the paper. I handed it in and returned to my medical rounds to wait and wait...and wait. Days, weeks, and months passed, and still I heard nothing from the doctor. Finally the waiting became too much. I asked the doctor how he was progressing on my thesis, on our thesis.

This drew a rare smile.

"My dear young friend," he said. "You are so young for a PhD thesis. You should not worry. At this stage in your career, you have a lot of time."

I was quiet, but couldn't help thinking that at this pace I would soon be too old for a PhD thesis. The paper finally appeared with the doctor's corrections, most of which were focused on punctuation and grammar. (He was editor of a major orthopedics journal and had the same tolerance for misplaced commas as he did for mis-placed sutures.)

The work was copied and bound into five hardcover books, one for each of the five "internal" reviewers who would have several weeks to scrutinize it before calling me in for a formal meeting to defend the doctoral thesis and display my knowledge of the specialty and related fields of medicine. I'd specialized in orthopedics. The questions that rained down on me were related to the effects of trauma, applications of microsurgery, the pathology of healing in vessels, the mechanics of thrombus formation, and the hemodynamics (the mechanisms of circulation) of the vascular system.

Then I waited.

The internal reviewers had three months to provide recommendations and determine whether the thesis was worthy of defense before the entire medical school. The thesis was also studied by two external reviewers to ensure that the university was not showing favoritism to its own when awarding degrees.

After what seemed like an eternity, the board announced that it had accepted the thesis. An announcement was duly published in the city's newspaper stating that I would be defending my thesis before the entire faculty of the medical school. The public was invited to attend, observe, and ask questions.

I made the presentation and responded to questions

from the doctors and the audience. I was asked to leave the room while the reviewers and senate deliberated and voted. When I was called back in, the dean of the school smiled at me, told me that the thesis had been unanimously accepted, and congratulated me on acquiring the degree of doctor of philosophy in orthopedics and microsurgery.

A few years later, after my fellowship in Louisville, I would make the same journey through the long night hours, the red ink, and the queries to present my dissertation, *Hemodynamics of the Microcirculation of the Free Muscle Flap in Experimental In Vivo Study,* and be awarded the degree of doctor of science for the work. The effort that time was familiar, but it wasn't that much easier.

I LEARNED MUCH about anatomy, biology, and hemodynamics in creating the two theses. Perhaps more important, these were my first forays into conducting basic research. At the time, the thought of conducting a face transplant never entered my mind, but as I digested red ink, I was learning the means and methods required to institute and accomplish such a procedure.

In light of the variety of organs, tissues, and structures that have already been transplanted from one individual to another, one has to wonder why a face transplant has not already been conducted. Hearts have been taken from one person and put into another, as have lungs, livers, kidneys, corneas, nerves, and a host of other organs and structures. Plastic surgeons have been remodeling the face for decades to restore dignity to the disfigured and beauty to the vain. So why not a face transplant?

There are two reasons, one technical and one biological. First, most restorative plastic surgery procedures being conducted today involve autografts — patches of skin, pieces of bone, and cartilage moved from one place on a patient's body to another. Since the patient's own tissues, cartilage, and bone are being used for the remodeling, there is no concern about immunological rejection.

Second, most of these procedures involve the remodeling of superficial tissues and/or structures that lie immediately beneath them. A patient whose face has been extensively damaged by fire or trauma may require a number of procedures because it is impossible to recover enough flesh from elsewhere on the person's body to cover the face with a single transfer.

Try this experiment. Put a large, damp napkin over your face and press it into all your features. The chances are good that it will take a major portion of that napkin to cover your face. Have a friend with a marker draw a line on the napkin starting about where the throat meets your chin. Continue the line around the back of your ear and over your forehead, following the hairline to the other ear and back to the starting point. Lift the napkin, smooth it out, and trim it along the line. Place it over various locations around your body and you will discover the difficulty surgeons have in finding enough skin to cover a face.

A complete or partial facial restoration thus requires the transfer of a number of patches of flesh over an extended period of time. While these may improve a person's features, the results seldom bring complete restoration to either appearance or function. When two pieces of flesh are joined, no matter how skilled the surgeon, no matter how fine the sutures, there will be scarring.

Scarring is natural and unavoidable. The scars may be all but invisible, but they'll be there, giving the juncture a certain rigidity. Moreover, the muscles and the nerves that control features of the face cannot be transferred with the sections of flesh to be grafted. The structure of abdominal muscles is completely different from those controlling the face. It would be futile to move them.

Therefore, patients whose faces have been extensively restored have faces that are essentially masks. They are incapable of expression, incapable of registering emotion, incapable of offering even the slightest smile to a child.

One of the promises of total face transplantation is

that the attachment of tissue to the facial muscles that lie beneath may restore a certain degree of control and function. Scarring will be limited to the periphery of the tissue (comparable to the outer edges of the trimmed napkin). The restoration of both appearance and a degree of function is one of the primary arguments in support of a full face transplant.

As the procedure is currently envisioned, the tissue and structures to be transplanted would be removed by an incision that circles the donor's entire face from the hairline at the scalp to well beneath the chin and back again. Hundreds of minute veins, arteries, and nerves will lie at the boundaries of the allograft. Although features may differ extensively from one person to another, the anatomy that allows them to function is reasonably similar. The veins, arteries, and nerves from the borders of the donor's face should match up closely with the same veins, arteries, and nerves on the recipient's face.

Joining these minute arteries, veins, and nerves constitutes the technical challenge. The resolution of this challenge began at the end of the 19th century, when the young Dr. Carrel first began visiting the seamstresses of Lyon to learn techniques that would allow him to suture ever-smaller veins.

The veins he sutured were 2 to 3 millimeters. The

size of veins being sutured has been growing smaller ever since. In 1960, Jules Jacobsen at the University of Vermont described the anastomosis of veins as small as 1.4 mm, which he accomplished using a microscope. Four years later Dr. Harry Buncke, working with rabbits' ears in a garage in California, rejoined vessels as small as 1 millimeter. Today, vessels half that size or smaller are being joined.

As technology advances, the vessels grow smaller, the sutures grow smaller, and the microscopes grow larger and more powerful. For instance, the diameters of suture thread used in conventional operations range from 0.07 to .3 mm. Sutures used in microsurgery may be as small as 0.05 to 0.1 mm. A grain of salt or a human hair may be 0.04 mm. This is close to the smallest structure an unaided eye can see. Microsurgery needles are only slightly larger than the sutures.

With the development of these sutures, needles, and other microsurgical instruments as well as the creation of microscopes dedicated to microsurgery, the technical challenge of face transplants has been largely overcome. As this book is being written, there are at least five surgical teams in the United States, France, the United Kingdom, and China that have the tools, skills, and experience to transplant a face.

The first hand transplants (which took place in France in 1998 and shortly thereafter in Louisville in 1999) and the first laryngeal transplant (performed in Cleveland in 1998) were landmark procedures for several reasons. First, they were significant surgical accomplishments. Second, they were among the first composite-tissue allografts. Unlike whole-organ transplants, these procedures included the successful transplantation of bone, muscles, tendons, nerves, and a mixture of tissues, which then regained a significant degree of function once healing was complete. Since then, there have been thigh- and knee-bone transplantations, at least four double hand transplants, a tongue transplant, and an abdominal wall transplant.

These procedures have also shown that the right combination of immunosuppressant drugs can prevent the complicated and extensive immune response that is to be expected when a variety of foreign tissues are brought together. This is the biological challenge. Immunological rejection is of course a concern in a heart transplant, but the tissues involved are relatively uniform. A face transplant involves a variety of tissues, and the host's immunological response, if not quelled, would be complex and powerful.

Different tissues prompt different degrees of immune responses. The emphasis here is placed on the term *degrees*.

Bear in mind that different tissues are not being joined. The layers of skin and ligaments to be transplanted will be joined to the recipient so each layer of skin meets its opposite. (Picture halves of two different layer cakes being brought together.) However, some tissues can be more immunologically reactive (immunogenic) than others. For instance, skin can harbor concentrations of dendritic cells. These powerful cells patrol the vasculature (blood vessels), and when they meet foreign cells or substances, one of their several actions is the release of potent cytokines, proteins that increase or upregulate the entire immune response by calling other immune cells to action.

Developing new immunosuppressive agents, combinations, and strategies is one of my primary areas of research. The goal is to create an immunological treatment that specifically hinders tissue rejection while permitting other immune responses to go on and minimizing side effects. In light of the complexity of the immune system, this is a significant challenge, but one that I am confident will be met, if not by researchers in my laboratory, then by someone else.

The varieties of transplant procedures that have become routine today show that immunosuppressive therapies are effective and can prevent tissue rejection. Without such certainty, a face transplant would not be conceivable. The technical and biological challenges have been met. Both may be improved as we move ahead, but at this moment in the history of medicine, our technical skill and biological ability are more than sufficient.

CHAPTER 7

Louisville Fellows

I GOT OFF THE plane in Louisville at the end of June 1985. After hours of breathing the stale air-conditioning of planes and airports, I walked outside under the open sky of Bluegrass country and felt as if I were diving into an aquarium left too long in the sun. I was prepared to learn medicine. I was prepared to spend the next several years of my life in America. I was prepared to meet new colleagues and make new friends. I was not prepared for a Kentucky summer.

I was also unprepared for the pace of American life. Dr. Ellen Beatty, then a young surgical fellow like myself (now a practicing hand surgeon in Tampa), met me at the plane with a smile, a handshake, and the news that I was on call at Jewish Hospital the next morning.

My shift started at 6 a.m., a time when the streets between my downtown apartment in the Kentucky Towers and the Jewish Hospital were still quiet, even a little sinister. Since then I've traveled the world many times over and found that it seems to be a general rule that no one ever builds a hospital in the best part of town.

The moment I walked onto the clinic floor, the world changed. It was as if I'd kicked over a beehive of angry acronyms.

Doctors and scientists from every non-English-speaking nation in the world have little trouble with the English language as it pertains to their specialty because they learn many medical and scientific terms early in their education. Many of the advanced texts are in English, and even if the language isn't dominant in conferences and symposia, it fills the halls outside the meeting rooms.

Nonetheless I was wholly unprepared for the shower of abbreviations that fell on me.

There were the OR, ER (emergency room), FDS (flexor digitorum sublimis tendon), and FDP (flexor digitorum profundus tendon), just for a sample. It was as if American medical specialists had for some reason abandoned their language altogether in favor of speaking in letters. Go to your computer and search "medical acronyms." You'll see dozens upon dozens of websites, some of which display up to 200,000 abbreviations and terms.

But the acronyms were only spice. The work was the meat, and there was a lot of it. Monday through Saturday, the day began with a 6 a.m. lecture. Sundays were easier. They started at 7 a.m. After lectures, we'd go into the hospital wards to make rounds. When we weren't in lectures, making rounds, or seeing patients in clinics, we were in surgery. The average day would end sometime between 10 p.m. and midnight. We spent about five days a week in surgery, and it was common to conduct seven or more procedures a day.

This surgical workload may seem surprising for a specialty clinic located in Kentucky, but remember, this is the heart of farm country. My theory is that what kept us surgeons so busy was the profound love Americans have for machines.

An American farm is nearly as mechanized as an American factory. Our patients, mostly men, were either unfamiliar with their new machines or perhaps too familiar with their old ones. The result was that gears, blades, belts, wheels, pulleys, and all the other moving parts seemed to be constantly attacking the men who used them.

Throughout the Midwest, the Louisville center was known for its expertise. Louisville's citizens were so familiar with the thump and throb of life-flight helicopters rushing patients in from distant cities and counties that they hardly noticed when one passed overhead.

The work fell heavily on the fellows. We were on call eight to ten times a month. So in addition to performing our standard duties of caring for patients and performing scheduled surgeries, we had to be ready to respond to any call coming from the emergency room.

There were three levels of "on-call" status. If you were on the first list, you had to remain in the hospital, ready to get to the emergency room when a patient arrived, if not before. Second-level on-call surgical fellows might be able to go home as long as they remained tied to a beeper. Third-level fellows served as backups to the backups.

The faculty of the hand institute brought organization to the mayhem. At the time, these surgeons, among the most remarkable I've ever met, were Dr. Harold Kleinert, Dr. Joseph Kutz, Dr. Erdogan Atasoy, Dr. Thomas Wolff, Dr. Tsu-Min Tsai, and Dr. Graham Lister. The eight or so fellows at the institute would serve a rotation under each of these men. It would have been wonderful to have had these men all to ourselves. However, their reputations were such that they drew residents from the school and surgeons from around the nation and the world.

It was often difficult for us to follow them, for each

of these surgeons had a different approach to the same procedures. Yet each produced spectacular results. At the close of every rotation, the faculty member leading the training would take his motley crowd of fellows out to dinner at a local restaurant. Except for Dr. Kleinert. He offered the fellows a home-cooked country meal at his farm across the border in Indiana, giving young physicians from all over the world the experience of a down-home dinner.

Dr. Harold Kleinert is a thin, tall, bright-eyed man who favors bow ties. A pack rat, he's one of those men who never lets go of anything he touches or anything that touches him. He has never sold a car he bought or passed up a chance to buy an antique car he fancied.

When I visited his farm, Dr. Kleinert's barn was empty of cows but full of cars — enough to fill a modest-sized downtown parking lot. And there probably wouldn't have been room left on the lot for his collection of antique farm machinery and implements. His beautifully restored farmhouse also included a room filled wall-to-wall with antique dolls.

Any trip to the farm involved a tour of these odd collections. Since the fellowship began, more than 900 young doctors have rotated through the institute, exploring the Kleinert farm, barn, cars, and dolls. That's a lot of steak, chops, chicken, and corn on the cob — and a lot of young people from other lands wondering about the function of that strange but wonderfully preserved piece of bright green machinery sitting in the corner of the barn.

Dr. Kleinert founded the University of Louisville Hand Clinic in 1953 and was joined five years later by Dr. Kutz. These two men were legendary hand surgeons then and remain so today. Dr. Kutz is a big man with large hands that can perform amazingly delicate microsurgical procedures. It was and still is the doctors' reputation that draws so many other noted surgeons to the clinic.

When I was at the hand clinic, Dr. Lister was the only member of the team who did not have the letters MD following his name. Instead, he proudly displayed FRCS, which stood for Fellow of the Royal College of Surgeons, a reminder of his Scottish roots. He ran the fellowship program with the sort of organization and demand for punctuality usually reserved for a railway stationmaster in Scotland.

I think of Tsu-Min Tsai as the perfect microsurgeon, a man with a remarkable ability to replant severed hands, fingers, toes, and thumbs. At the time, fellows rotating under Dr. Tsai had another responsibility: despite his many years in the U.S., he retained a thick accent, and fellows standing at the patient's bedside often had to act as translators. Picture a young fellow from Poland, standing next to a world-renowned Taiwanese surgeon, explaining a procedure to a Kentucky farmer with a drawl as thick as butter.

Dr. Atasoy graduated from the University of Istanbul in Turkey. He specialized in nerve compression in the head and neck, pioneering procedures to relieve thoracic outlet compression syndrome, a painful neck problem involving the muscles tied to the first rib and backbone.

Dr. Wolff is what every kid outside the U.S. imagines an American to be. When I worked with him, he was easygoing, always laughing and joking—and the fastest microsurgeon I've ever scrubbed in with.

And then there were the fellows, young surgeons from Japan, China, Argentina, Peru, Germany, Norway, Canada, Israel, the U.S., South Africa, and Poland, all of whom spoke English passably and medicine excellently. Together we got through the long days of coffee in paper cups, people in need, and lectures on the secrets of putting flesh and bone, muscle and nerve back together. We laughed at our experiences with the strange American culture and commiserated with each other when mistakes were made. We worked shoulder to shoulder for hours on end, bent over mutilated hands, arms, legs, and toes. We learned and became friends, and then we became a family.

A snapshot of all of us — faculty and fellows, old and young, men and women, our faces reflecting every race and culture on the planet — would be a picture of the practice of medicine as it was evolving at the close of the 20th century and into the 21st. Walk the corridors of any hospital almost anywhere in the world and you'll see men and women of every nationality hurrying toward a patient's room. You'll see them reviewing a chart at the nurses' station or gathered over coffee in a corner, speculating on the origin of a patient's fever, the outcome of tonight's basketball game, or tomorrow's menu in the cafeteria. I can think of no other profession so unconstrained by race, gender, religion, nationality, or politics. Medicine is unique.

FOR EVERY PLACE I've been and for any given span of time, there has been a clinical case that stands as fresh in my mind as if it happened just hours ago. There were two such in Kentucky.

The first is emblematic of the teamwork, determination, and patience that challenging medical procedures demand of those who conduct them. The second is an example of the ethical challenges doctors face, sometimes on a daily basis, when they have to weigh the balance between risk and benefit while listening to the inner voice of clinical experience, the one that tells them they can go this far and no farther — even when they know their skills might, just might, produce a significantly better outcome. It's a place that lies somewhere between "I think I can" and "I know I can." Finding it is not always easy.

I remember the first case well. The call came out to all the surgeons and fellows in the afternoon. A helicopter was bringing in an out-of-state patient who had severed all his fingers, four from one hand and four from the other. The fingers had been retrieved and we were to replace them.

Within minutes of the chopper touching down on the hospital roof, two teams of faculty and fellows, one for each hand, were at work. One was debriding the stumps on the hands, and the other was debriding the amputated fingers.

Fingers, like all moving parts of the human anatomy, are wonderfully engineered, tremendously complicated structures. One anatomy text devotes ten pages of illustrations to identifying the structures of the hand and fingers. Identifying the fine structures of the hand — the nerves, arteries, veins, tendons, and varied layers of flesh and muscle — would probably fill another two dozen pages.

It's curious how time suspends itself when you're concentrating. When you bend into the eyepieces of a surgical microscope, the world outside the small circle of tissue in the view disappears. Time stops. Progress is measured by sutures as they are placed one after another into the tiny arteries and veins encompassed by the circle. I may have remained bent over a finger for perhaps three hours or longer before standing and backing away from the operating table to stretch.

We fell into an unspoken rhythm. One by one we'd rise, stretch, step outside the OR to go to the bathroom or swallow a cup of coffee before putting on new gowns and masks, scrubbing, and stepping back inside. The operation began late in the afternoon and continued through the night.

The next morning the second shift came into the OR to be briefed on the procedure's progress and take over. I can remember looking over my shoulder as I left. Several fingers remained to be reattached, but those that were in place were already pink. I think this is how mountain climbers must feel when they reach the top of some great peak: wholly rewarded, wholly satisfied, and completely exhausted.

The second case was just as memorable. The patient was twenty-three. It was Christmas Eve. She was brought into the hospital with both legs amputated. A railroad train had taken them off just below the knee.

A railroad train wheel is a huge, ugly blunt instrument. It doesn't cut like a knife so much as it severs by crushing, the way you would a peeled banana if you squeezed it between your thumb and forefinger. The routine in replantations is to evaluate both stump and limb to assess the damage to each and to determine what can be cleaned, what can be preserved, what can be restored, and what must be discarded.

The damage in this instance was extensive, especially to the bones in the severed legs. An accurate evaluation of the integrity of these bones was especially important, since if they were rescued they would serve as the foundation and scaffolding for the restoration. The attending physicians and fellows pored over the X-rays of the young woman's limbs. Other surgeons were called and told to abandon their holiday celebrations and come to the hospital.

The discussion that followed was similar to those that transpire in hospitals around the world every day: *What do we know we can do? What do we think we can do? What should we try? When is conservative too conservative? Where is that fine line between acceptable and unacceptable risk?* There are no definitive answers to these questions, but they must be answered — and answered while the clock is running. We may not know for days, months, or years whether the answers are right or wrong. We may never know.

We determined almost immediately that the bones that were to serve as the "bridges" were far too damaged to permit the legs to be reattached. Bridges are those sections of bone and tissue that are to be joined. It was a tough decision for highly experienced surgeons to make and an even tougher one to impose on a beautiful young woman just beginning to shape her life. The decision to forgo attempts at reattachment spawned a host of other clinical decisions.

We wanted to preserve and reconstruct as much of the bone and tissue below the knee as possible. This was terribly important and no small challenge. If her legs were to be amputated above the knee, her eventual gait would always involve an obvious lurch and thrust, even with the most advanced prosthetic legs. If we could preserve the knee joint and something of the bone below it, the right prosthesis and rehabilitation might allow her stride to appear normal.

We recovered arteries, veins, and tissue from the amputated legs, using them to reconstruct as much as possible of the young woman's legs below the knee. Although we were not able to reattach the legs, the results of our work left a young woman with a far better life than she might have had if she had suffered her accident at any great distance from one of the world's renowned microsurgical centers.

The first case, the man who had severed his fingers, presented no ethical problems. We knew what could be done and we did it. On the other hand, the young woman's clinical circumstances raised a number of recurring ethical issues. She was surrounded by a host of skilled surgeons, all of whom wanted to push their abilities as far as they could to get the best possible results for the patient.

But the farther you reach beyond what you are absolutely certain can be done, the farther you move into an unknown where rewards and risks are not well defined. How much risk can you ask a patient to accept? How well can you educate a person about the risks involved when that person may have no greater understanding of biology than what she learned in a high school science class? How much trust can you put in the decision of a traumatized young patient who desperately wants her life to be whole again, is terribly frightened of a future she cannot imagine, and may be willing to accept any risk as long as it contains a glimmer of hope?

This last question reflects one of the greatest changes that medicine has undergone in the 20th century. The challenge of balancing anticipated rewards against estimated risks reaches back to the origins of the profession. Allowing the patient to weigh these factors and make the final decision is a new idea, one that your grandparents never considered, even if they were physicians.

My first vague desire to transplant a face arose in Louisville. Farm machinery mutilated many hands. Fire damaged others. But burns are seldom limited to hands. Fire is an all-consuming beast, and the patients we saw with damaged hands usually suffered extensive burn damage to their bodies, including their faces. My colleagues and I could restore function to hands, and the damage to the trunk and arms could be covered by clothes. But those who suffered extensive damage to their faces would forever be socially crippled in a society that appears to value beauty above all other human characteristics.

At that time, when the first vague considerations of a face transplant began to take form in my mind, I had no idea of the issues involved. I was to learn that one of the greater challenges to performing a face transplant lay not in the sterile conditions of the OR but in the offices of medical ethicists in the United States and around the world.

My first research efforts in Louisville, however, were far from controversial. "We now report the development of a new cremaster muscle preparation," read a signature sentence in one of the first studies from Kentucky bearing my name as a coauthor. It appeared in a 1987 issue of the journal *Microvascular Research*, a magazine you're unlikely to find at your local newsstand.

I first met Dr. Robert Acland, professor of surgery at the University of Louisville, during the latter half of the 1980s when I worked as a fellow at the Institute for Hand and Microsurgery in Louisville. Dr. Acland, his colleagues, and I gave the microsurgical community a significantly improved model of the study of microcirculation.

Obviously, researchers do not begin to experiment with medicines or procedures in human beings until every other possible avenue is thoroughly explored. To do this, we design models of trauma and disease as any self-respecting craftsman would, replicating reality as closely as possible. If you want to find out how the *Titanic* sank, build an exact model of the great ship, tear a hole in its side, put it in water, observe closely, and take notes. If you want to find out how blood flows through a newly sutured 1 mm vein, get a rat muscle, isolate it, sever a vein, suture it, observe closely, and take notes.

The cremaster muscle is in the lower abdomen, covering the testicles in many mammals, including humans. It helps raise and lower the scrotum to control testicular temperature and preserve the viability of sperm. The virtue of this particular muscle is that it can be peeled away from an anesthetized animal and placed on a glass stage with a light below and a microscope above. The muscle is so thin that when the light is turned on, the view in the microscope is not unlike that from a traffic helicopter looking down on a busy interstate highway system. Every cell, every complex aspect of blood flow, tissue destruction, and repair appears before your eyes in real time like a movie unfolding.

Surgeons are a conservative crowd. We dislike surprises. As a matter of fact, we hate them with unbridled passion. Unexpected and unanticipated responses to our actions put knots in our stomachs.

Transplanting a free flap is a common procedure in plastic surgery. It involves acquiring a thicker slice of tissue, one that holds blood vessels, muscle, skin, and fat. This challenging procedure is used to reconstruct noses, breasts, and other structures. Nearly every surgeon has had an instance in which the procedure is moving along smoothly and nearing completion when suddenly the flap or a portion of it loses color.

In what seems like seconds, that wonderful shade of pink that signifies viability begins to move toward white or blue, indicating that blood flow is compromised or interrupted. If the tissue has a white cast, it suggests that the vessels affected are arteries. Blue indicates that the problem lies with veins.

The surgeon's first thought is that the anastomoses, the junctures where the flap's vessels have been sutured to the receiving vessels, have become compromised. A thrombus, a clot, has formed to obstruct blood flow. The vessels may have become twisted or kinked like a mistreated garden hose as the flap was being maneuvered and fixed into place.

The mystery deepens when inspection of these potential defects shows the vessels to be perfectly clear. It deepens even more when just as suddenly as the problem appeared, it disappears. For reasons unknown the flap resumes a shade of living pink as venous outflow returns. This is accompanied by relief among the members of the operating team and a sense of frustration that lasts long after everyone has scrubbed out and is sitting around sipping the sort of bad coffee that can only be found in hospital cafeterias after hours. Although the problem resolved itself, it was an unwelcome surprise. The surgical team wants to know what happened and, more importantly, why.

Our Kentucky rat-cremaster model offered some tentative answers to the origins of the phenomenon. When blood flow to a flap is interrupted by a scalpel and restored by suturing donor vessels to recipient vessels to create the juncture called an anastomosis, numerous small clumps — emboli — form in the lumen, the interior of the vessel. These float in the blood, looking like socks filled with pudding. These emboli appear suddenly, grow in number, and just as suddenly fade away. We called the phenomenon an "embolic storm." In most instances, this swell of emboli moves through the vasculature easily, but where small vessels split into even smaller vessels, the emboli slow and get hung up on the sharp edge of the split. As we stated in our study:

> *On one occasion we were able to follow the fate of an embolus as it traveled through the arteriolar branching system.... As the embolus progressed from larger to smaller vessels, its shape changed from a fat blob to a long, thin cord that quite filled the vessel it was moving in. At each bifurcation that it came to, the embolus was driven into one or the other branch, stayed there motionless for 5 to 30 seconds, and then suddenly moved on, each time smaller than before.*

This is another aspect of research rarely mentioned: A researcher seeing these events for the first time may feel like Lewis and Clark standing on a high ridge west of the Missouri, looking into a valley never before seen by eyes from the east. The wonder of discovery can occur in medical research, tedious as that research might seem when it involves staring through a microscope at tissue from a rat scrotum. Every once in a while we get to say, "Wow!"

I gained a number of valuable insights into biological systems in Dr. Acland's laboratory and — just as important — I learned that good research must not only be good but also look good. The laboratories you see in the movies too often look like something you'd find at a scientific garage sale. Machines whir and wink, displays flicker, and fluids bubble through a maze of glass pipes. It may heighten the drama, but it's inaccurate.

In a laboratory actively pursuing scientific discovery — and especially in Dr. Acland's laboratory — each piece of equipment is placed precisely according to its purpose and function. There is no extraneous material nearby, no nest of test tubes or pile of petri dishes, and there are no whirrs, winks, flickers, or bubbles. The design and progress of the experiment are apparent even to the untrained eye. Photographs of the experimental setup and subsequent results are always in focus, always uncluttered, always well-lit and composed.

This is how science should be done. This is how elegant experiments are designed. This is how unquestioned discoveries are made.

To this day, I believe that I am truly fortunate to be able to conduct research and practice medicine simultaneously. The great majority of practicing physicians have little opportunity to pursue research. They're simply too busy. They also lack the funding and facilities to conduct proper investigations. Laboratories and equipment are expensive. Even more important, such labs require skilled technicians to maintain them and a constant flow of fellows and research assistants to give life to the lab. They come to the lab bench with open minds and fresh eyes. They ask new questions and offer new perspectives.

Some laboratories are dominated by a principal researcher who asks the questions and figures out how to get the answers. Maria Sklodowska of Warsaw, better known as Madame Marie Curie, was one of these. But in most labs advances result from collaboration between eager and energetic young fellows pursuing inquiries and an experienced principal investigator offering direction.

Research taught me not only to always ask questions but also to ask them in a way that suggests a path to an answer. This approach to medicine, acquired through years of research, is an invaluable benefit at the bedside.

When something isn't going right — when a graft isn't healing as it should, when a fever persists, when there is pain when there shouldn't be — the ability to ask the right questions and to frame them so that they produce answers that can be applied is a skill to be sought and refined. When the right questions are asked in the laboratory, the answers become part of a clinician's working knowledge and art. When you see tissue responding to this stimulus or that stimulus under a microscope in a laboratory, you can then look at a wound in a patient and see the same microscopic events in your mind's eye. A microscope is unnecessary. You know what's happening and what to do about it.

I've worked with and trained many bright, talented young medical students, and too often I am disappointed to find that they seem to have lost the ability to ask sound clinical questions. I'm not talking about the questions they ask their patients or the questions they ask their mentors, but the questions that they should be asking of the biological systems they see beneath the lens of a microscope. They don't ask the questions that would allow them to make the leap from the microscope to the bedside. They don't ask the questions that allow them to say "Wow!"

෧෨

CHAPTER 8

Transplants

THE BERLIN WALL fell in 1989. I was in Louisville at the time, but just like Poles and Eastern Europeans everywhere, I heard the crash loud and wonderfully clear. The Wall fell during my second visit to Louisville.

My first visit to Louisville and the United States was in 1985. Taking a career step into a new institution in a new city in a new nation was a challenge, so Vlodek and I decided to take smaller steps rather than one large one. I went first and scouted the area, and then Vlodek and Kris followed six months later. The steps were perhaps small for my husband and me, but for Kris, it was a frightening leap. He had just entered school in Poland when he had to say goodbye to the new friends and fly across a great ocean to live in a new country.

The day after he arrived, still weary from his journey, he was enrolled in the second grade. His first day of school, I was on call and had to leave for the clinic at 6 a.m., before Kris left for school. I remember turning on the walk to see a small boy with a backpack sitting alone in the window, waiting for the school bus and a future in a strange nation that must have seemed larger than any child could have imagined.

Yet within three months, Kris was translating jokes for Vlodek and me. We spoke English but we couldn't speak it the way Kentuckians did. Kris could, and only he could translate the story about the farmer and the three-legged dog; more important, only he could tell us why it was really, really funny.

We returned to Poland for a while and went back to Louisville a year and a half later. This time, we made the jump together as a family and the hurdle wasn't nearly so high. Kris was bigger and stronger and now spoke English with little trace of an accent. From Louisville, we would leap to Salt Lake City and from Salt Lake City to Cleveland, Ohio. By the time we arrived in Ohio, Kris had soldiered through a number of private and public schools and had emerged with a high school diploma from Salt Lake City and a degree from Ohio University.

Today Kris sometimes stops by my office to say hello

when he's not too busy. He's in his last year of a six-year residency in orthopedics at Cleveland Clinic. I'm proud beyond words of his accomplishments as a young man and doctor, and even more impressed by the courage he displayed as a boy in a strange country where no one spoke his language. I have no idea how many dragons, imaginary and real, he must have slain to get to where he is now, but there must have been many, and some undoubtedly very large.

But when the Berlin Wall fell, my biggest dragons were alive and breathing fire.

In the late 1980s, Dr. Graham Lister, the surgeon who offered me a Louisville fellowship at the symposium in Yugoslavia years earlier, accepted a position as Chairman of the Department of Plastic Surgery at the University of Utah School of Medicine in Salt Lake City. He called and asked whether I would like to be director of the Division of Plastic Surgery Research. There was one drawback: there was no Division of Plastic Surgery Research. I would have to set it up.

It was an offer I couldn't refuse. My husband, son, and I arrived in Salt Lake City in 1990. The university gave me seed money to establish a lab equal to the task of attracting fellows from around the world and provided the resources to offer up to 40 hours of continuing medical education courses in microsurgery to the area's surgeons.

In the winter, when it gets cold in Louisville, people tend to stay inside. In Salt Lake City, people look forward to winter sports. They stay outside — sometimes too long. Our ER saw plenty of frostbite cases.

Cold can be an ally or an enemy. Frostbite and the effects of cold on tissue and circulation still hold some mysteries. When cold settles on the stranded snowboarder who lost his gloves during the last tumble, blood vessels begin to constrict, nerves deaden, skin temperature falls, blood vessels freeze, and ice crystals form around and within cells. Ischemia (the cessation of blood flow) deprives cells of oxygen, and if the condition persists, cells perish. This is why organs scheduled for transplant are rushed so quickly from donor to recipient. The hand of the Finnish woodchopper was not dead and preserved like a pork chop or steak; its cells were very much alive. The ice was slowing the rate at which those cells burned what energy stores remained within their walls in the absence of replenishment by a working circulatory system.

The clock starts when blood stops flowing to a cell, a tissue, or an organ. When the temperature of that cell, tissue, or organ is lowered (a process called hypothermia) the clock slows down. Cooling tissue to be transplanted is a way of buying extra time. But how much extra time does hypothermia buy? And by what mechanism does it do so?

One of the research findings we made in Salt Lake City is that in addition to prolonging a tissue's lifespan, hypothermia also assists its acceptance in a new location by reducing or eliminating leukocytes, better known as white blood cells. These cells are central to the immune system's inflammatory response.

This response is normally a good thing, but if you are transplanting tissue, even autologous tissue (not derived from anyone or anything other than the patient), from one area of a patient to another, the last thing you want is leukocytes initiating inflammation in the microcirculatory system. We discovered that one reason cooling tissue preserves its viability and reduces inflammation is that leukocytes are temperature-sensitive. This observation — that cold reduces or eliminates leukocytes from transplanted tissue and thus reduces the opportunity for inflammation — illustrates the fact that for the most part medical science doesn't advance breakthrough by breakthrough, but bit by bit. The leukocyte finding was just one piece of an extremely large and complicated medical puzzle that continues to be studied.

It was in Salt Lake City that I started on the path that

would eventually lead me to propose a face transplant. At this point in medical history, a host of surgeons around the world and I had the skills necessary to complete the physical tasks that the procedure involved. What we didn't have was the ability to overcome the recipient's immune response. I began my first attempts to control that response in Salt Lake City.

THE IMMUNE SYSTEM is not an organ but an army of different cells, each of which has differing responsibilities and weapons. Identifying those cells, their functions, and their means of communication has occupied medical science since the end of the 18th century and continues to perplex us today, even though we now have tools that allow us to discern and describe the structure, not of cells, but of molecules on the surface of cells.

Touch a thorn to flesh and you will trigger one of the most powerful biological forces known. The human immune system defies description. It's quick, exquisitely sensitive, complex, and subtle. It's versatile, comprehensive, and durable. It never forgets, and it's seldom deceived. It's everyone's ally — and it's the biggest challenge a transplant surgeon and her patients face. That challenge is particularly substantial when the transplant involves a composite-tissue allograft (different type of tissues transplanted in one component from other people). But the challenge can be overcome.

The picture we have today of the immune system was assembled like a jigsaw puzzle, piece by piece, during the last two centuries. There was no steady pace to these discoveries. Medical science, as does all other science, progresses in fits and starts.

If a date can be set for the discovery of the first piece of the puzzle, most would say that it would be 1796.

That year, a 26-year-old French army officer named Bonaparte married an older woman named Joséphine de Beauharnais, George Washington's farewell address to the newborn United States was published in Philadelphia newspapers, and in Berkeley, England, a country physician named Edward Jenner extracted fluid from a milkmaid's cowpox sores and dribbled it into cuts on the arm of a farm boy named James Phipps. Six weeks later, the doctor made small cuts on the boy's arm and poured in fluid known to contain the highly contagious and often-deadly smallpox virus. Aside from being irritated about being fussed over by a doctor, the lad was unaffected. He had been rendered immune.

Phipps was certainly not the first to be "vaccinated," a term Dr. Jenner coined from *vacca*, the Latin word for cow. Others before Jenner had tried exposing patients to smallpox, but invariably they had used virulent strains. Some of those patients became immune to the disease. Others were buried.

What set Dr. Jenner apart from his colleagues was that he approached the procedure scientifically. He noted that farmhands and milkmaids exposed to cowpox developed sores and blisters, but seldom did the symptoms become worse. As he wandered the countryside treating patients, he also observed that men and women exposed to cowpox didn't seem to develop smallpox. He developed a theory and tested it on young Phipps.

Two years later, Dr. Jenner took the study one step further. He published his results and was promptly and resoundingly ridiculed by most of the medical community. This pattern — observation, theory, experiment, analysis, conclusion, and publication — is the essence of scientific method. (Ridicule is not, but it still occurs on occasion.)

Dr. Jenner was not the first to identify an immune response. Centuries before, physicians had noted that transplanted tissue was invariably rejected when the tissue was not autologous. What Dr. Jenner did, in addition to developing a means of combating a dread disease afflicting mankind, was to show that the immune system could be manipulated, that it could be taught to combat disease.

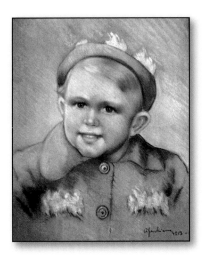

*This portrait of me, painted in 1953
by A. Frankiewicz, adorned a wall
in my home for years.*

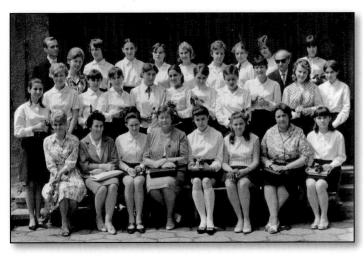

*My high school class photo: Young women ready and eager to
face the world. I'm in the top row, sixth from the left.*

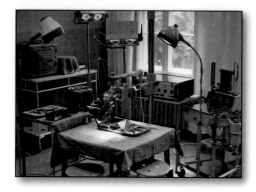

My first microsurgical laboratory was located in what used to be a Carmelite cloister. It is now the Hand Surgery Clinic in the Institute of Orthopaedics and Rehabilitation, University of Medical Sciences, Poznan.

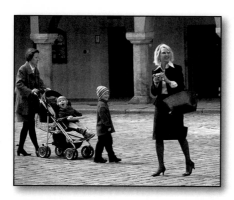

That's me with a camera, acting like a tourist in my hometown, while two blasé young inhabitants look on.

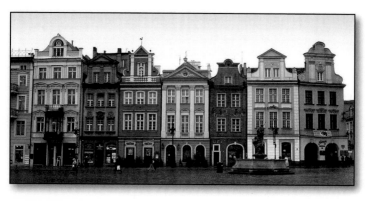

Established more than three centuries before Columbus discovered the New World, Poznan Old Market has been bustling with commerce for more than 700 years.

In 1974, I earned my medical degree after six long years.

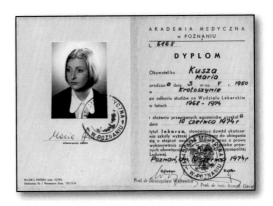

Wlodzimierz Siemionow and I were married at the town hall April 27, 1975.

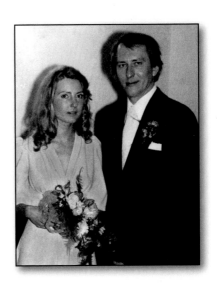

My doctoral thesis, from which the illustration is taken, focused on how to employ variations of Dr. Alexis Carrel's triangle method in the repair of blood vessels smaller than 1 mm.

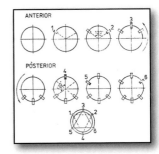

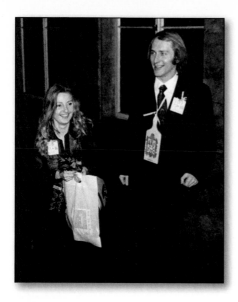

Senior Alumni Ball, 1976: The Bal Senior is an annual event drawing alumni from all of Poznan's universities.

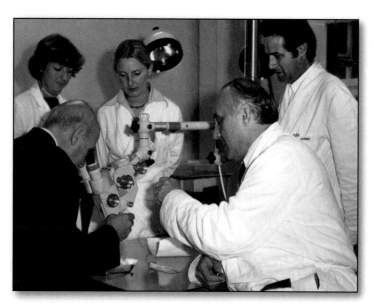

Victor Krylov, father of Russian microsurgery, peers through a microscope designed for microsurgerical studies during a 1978 visit to our department. To his right is Professor Dr. Strzyewski, Chairman of the Hand Surgery and Microsurgery Department, University of Medical Sciences, Poznan. Flanked by two colleagues, I watch from across the table.

Italian surgeon Gaspare Tagliocozzi transplanted skin from patients' own inner arms to recreate their mutilated noses (Italy, 1746). It is safe to assume that the procedure was extremely uncomfortable at best.

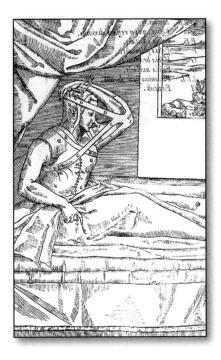

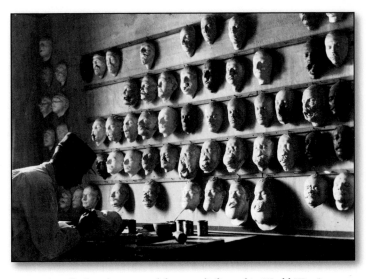

A wall of masks prepared for men disfigured in World War I. They were called "airman masks" because pilots often suffered horrible disfiguring burns when their planes were shot down.

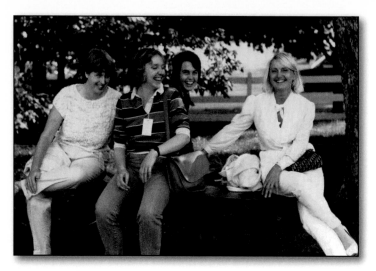

Fellows of Christine Kleinert Institute of Hand and Microsurgery Clinic in Louisville in the summer of 1985. From left: Barbara LeBlanc, Kay Kirkpatrick, Ellen Beatty, and me. It was a milestone year, the first in which the clinic could boast of so many female microsurgeons.

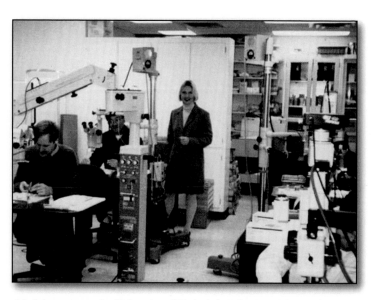

My laboratory at the University of Utah, Salt Lake City. This is where my microsurgery fellows worked and learned new techniques. Two of the main topics of study were microcirculation and transplantation.

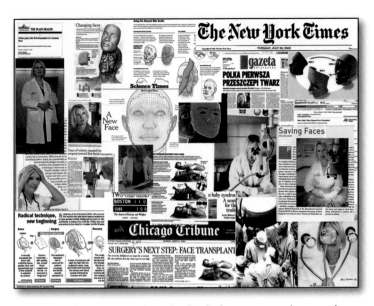

The media response. When Cleveland Clinic announced approval of a plan for a full face transplant in November 2004.

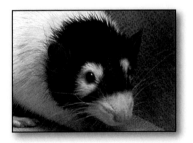

Zorro, so-called for obvious reasons, is a very special animal. The dark mask is a transplant from another rat. The transplanted tissue has survived without rejection for more than two years. Immunosuppressants were administered for only a short period following the transplant. This animal holds the promise that someday transplants may occur under a brief therapeutic protocol that eliminates the need for lifelong immunosuppressant.

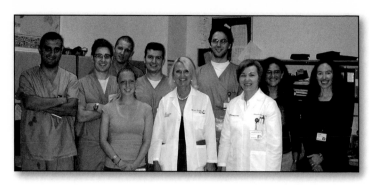

*This picture from 2007 shows me with my microsurgery
surgical fellows in the Microsurgery Laboratory at Cleveland Clinic.
From left: Serdar Nasir (Turkey), William Dugan (Ireland),
Lukasz Krokowicz (Poland), Christopher Grykien (Netherlands),
and Erhan Sonmez (Turkey). Front row: student Jill Froimson,
me, Aleksandra Klimczak (Poland), Jennifer Mule, and
Tracy Folger, my administrative assistant.*

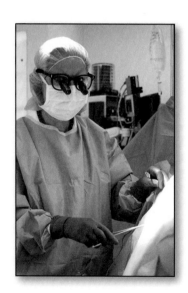

*In surgery. The glasses I am wearing
are called surgical loupes. They
are essential in microsurgerical
procedures and are custom-made
for each surgeon. As the hours pass,
they seem to become ever heavier.*

*Dr. Krzysztof (Kris) Siemionow.
Kris is an orthopaedic resident
at Cleveland Clinic. He plans to
specialize in spine surgery.*

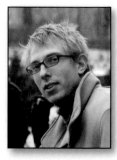

It was a start.

For nearly a century after Jenner's discoveries, a span stretching from the 1780s to the 1890s, advances in the understanding of the immune system were few. Then as the 20th century dawned, a remarkable crop of discoveries blossomed. The meaning of some of these discoveries was immediately apparent. The meaning of others would remain obscure for half a century or longer.

Robert Koch, one of the giants of medicine, started things rolling. During a professional career spanning 50 years, the doctor made significant advances in understanding anthrax, cholera, tuberculosis, diphtheria, malaria, blackwater fever, and typhus, among other diseases. It was Dr. Koch's assistant, Julius Richard Petri, who created the flat, shallow dish familiar to every youth who has taken a high school biology course. Because of this simple creation, Petri and his dish are probably more familiar to the world in general than Dr. Koch, a Nobel Prize winner. One of the doctor's contributions was the recognition of delayed hypersensitivity, the ability of the immune system to respond more rapidly to the second exposure to a pathogen or toxin than to the first. His observation suggests that the immune system has a memory.

Dr. Paul Ehrlich, a colleague of Koch's, was the sort of scientist Hollywood would love. Ideas assaulted him unexpectedly day and night, and when they did, he would scribble them on any available surface: walls, tabletops, napkins, his shirt cuffs, and presumably his assistants if they stood still for too long.

Dr. Ehrlich maintained that it was toxins released by cells, not necessarily the cells themselves, that destroyed pathogens. This was known as humoral immunity. The term was derived from the ancient view that all illness resulted from an imbalance of the four humors — yellow bile, black bile, phlegm, and blood. The humors in turn were related to the four elements — earth, air, fire, and water.

Elie Metchnikoff, a Russian-born researcher working at the Pasteur Institute in Paris, published extensive studies showing that the immune system harbored cells that were the equivalent of sharks. The cells were macrophages. (*Macro* means big; *phage* means eat.) This was a major observation. It laid the foundation for the concept of "cellular immunity," but the discovery was not fully appreciated. Unfortunately, science sometimes clings to theories the way society clings to fashions. The fashionable theory at the turn of the century belonged to Ehrlich. His theory of humoral immunity held sway for nearly half a century before it became accepted that both he and Metchnikoff were right. Humoral immunity is an essential component of cellular immunity, and vice versa. One functions in conjunction with the other, and both must be understood and moderated if a transplant of blood, tissues, or organs is to succeed.

In 1909, Karl Landsteiner was working as a prosector in the Wilhelminenspital in Vienna. A prosector is the individual who dissects and otherwise prepares cadavers for lectures and demonstrations given to medical students. Dr. Landsteiner recalled the work of a German named Leonard Landois, who described experiments in which the red corpuscles in animal blood clumped and eventually perished when placed in contact with human blood. The destruction of the cells released hemoglobin into the system. Dr. Landsteiner, who had a sharp eye for subtle biological activity, noted that the same thing sometimes happened when the blood of two individuals mixed. He surmised that the reaction might lead to the shock, jaundice, and hemoglobinuria (hemoglobin in urine) seen in attempts to transfuse blood. In 1909, he published a study that identified four fundamental groupings of human blood — A, B, AB, and O. He demonstrated that transfusion between some groups leads to disaster.

To this day, the immune system continues to astound and confound medical science. In its power, complexity, and versatility, it is rivaled only by the brain, yet the system is as nebulous as morning fog. It is everywhere and nowhere. The writer Gertrude Stein once said of Los Angeles, "There is no there there." The same could be said of the immune system. There's no central spot or organ one can point to and say, "There is the immune system." The system reaches from the surface of the skin to the deepest recesses of the heart. Wherever blood flows, the immune system follows, and blood reaches every living cell in the body.

Although there may be no "there" there, the system does have an origin. Most of the numerous types of cells in the system begin as stem cells in bone marrow. These evolve to one of three cell lineages: erythrocytes, which are red blood cells; megakaryocytes, which become platelets, the cells involved in clotting; and leukocytes, which after a few intermediary steps, become macrophages, neutrophils, eosinophils, basophils, dendritic cells, T-cells, B cells, and natural killer (NK) cells.

These cells have abilities that would shame a comic-book superhero. They can identify a single foreign cell among hundreds of thousands of cells. Not only will they attack and destroy that cell, but they will also alert and summon all their companions. They educate newly arrived immune cells about the character of the foreign cells, dispatching them through the system on a search-

and-destroy mission that won't stop until every foreign cell is reduced to harmless debris and expelled.

When all is done, the system returns to a state of quiet vigilance. It remembers forever the specific character of the foreign cell, and should that cell present itself a second time, the system's response will be so rapid that the foreign cell will never have the opportunity to establish a foothold.

In addition, there are three key noncellular components of the immune system: antigens, antibodies, and cytokines. This isn't a comprehensive list of the components of the immune system. But it's enough to allow a general description of the system's response to foreign tissue, demonstrate the challenge the system creates for surgeons transplanting tissue, and show how we can intervene.

One of the first dilemmas confronting researchers who explore the immune system is: How do cells, living entities no more than a few microns across, differentiate between self and other? How do they tell friend from foe? Why don't they devour and destroy everything in their path, friend and foe alike?

The fact is that a single macrophage or dendritic cell can easily and rapidly differentiate between a cell sharing its heritage and one that does not, between like cells that are healthy and those infected with a bacterium or virus.

Immune cells roaming the vasculature and encountering millions upon millions of cells can identify the one stranger in less time than it takes you to touch your nose. An immune cell such as a macrophage needs only to brush against a single foreign cell to spark an immune response.

To the untrained eye peering through a microscope, all cells look like miniature fried eggs. But our cells are as unique to us as our facial features. If we increased the microscope's magnification until it reached a power that allowed us to see molecules, we would see that cells display proteins on their surfaces that rise from the cell's outer membranes like a forest. These proteins are not only specific to the species but also specific to the person.

The individuality that each person displays on the surface goes all the way to the core, down into the constituent cells, into the nuclei, and onto a set of genes on chromosome 6 known as the MHC or major histocompatibility complex. These genes hold the codes that are translated into proteins called human leukocyte antigens (HLA), which are displayed on cell surfaces. These antigens are unique to you and allow the immune cells roving your blood system to differentiate between your cells and those of a stranger.

There are two classes of MHC. Class I MHC antigens,

displayed on most cells, fall into three groups: A, B, and DR. These are the groups specialists try to "match" in organ and tissue transplants.

Class II antigens are triggers. They are present only on the surface of immune-system cells. When foreign tissue enters the body, fragments of its cellular proteins are ingested by macrophages and other cells, broken into peptides (fragments), and displayed on the surface membranes along with Class II antigens. It's as if the Class II molecule is waving a wanted poster and saying, *Hey, we have an invader, and this is what it looks like!*

Who responds to this alert? Macrophages, neutrophils, dendritic cells, T-cells, B cells, cytotoxic T lymphocytes (CTLs), and NK cells. Macrophages linger in a variety of tissues. They're the system's sanitation department, spending most of their time consuming the cellular debris left by other cells that have perished. You may live for decades, but your cells don't. Cells in practically every tissue die and are replaced by new cells. It's the job of the macrophages to clean up the mess.

Macrophages ingest viruses, bacteria, cells infected by these pathogens, and most important, cells and cellular debris from transplanted tissue. Everything that goes into a macrophage is fragmented. Then, in addition to displaying foreign peptides on its surface, the macrophage undergoes a profound change. It sends out signals in the form of proteins called cytokines. Among these are interleukins (IL), interferons (INF), and tumor necrosis factor-alpha (TNF-a). When the macrophage releases these into the bloodstream, it's the equivalent of pouring blood into shark-infested waters. The cytokines activate other immune cells that begin to collect in the area the signals are emanating from.

Neutrophils (white blood cells), the most numerous cells in the bloodstream, are already at the site in substantial numbers. It's estimated that an adult creates ten billion neutrophils daily, a production that increases tenfold in the presence of infection. White blood cells are familiar to you as pus. These cells are particularly agile.

Endothelial cells, the cells that line the walls of blood vessels, are normally smooth, but in the presence of inflammation, endothelial cells extend molecules that make up a kind of biological Velcro. Each molecule snags a different type of immune cell. When the adhesion molecules link the cell to the wall of the endothelium, the cells undergo a transformation. They become remarkably plastic, able to slide between the cells lining the walls of the vessel and into infected or foreign tissue.

Dendritic cells are spread throughout the body from the skin to spaces between tissues to the lymph nodes. No matter where an infection erupts or tissue is transplanted, dendritic cells are there to identify and absorb the foreign antigens. These cells also respond to cytokines such as the tumor necrosis factor-alpha (TNF), which is secreted by activated macrophages. When activated, dendritic cells suddenly bristle with MHC II molecules like the raised quills on a porcupine. The cells begin to migrate and eventually reach the lymph nodes where they lodge, still bristling with MHC II and antigen.

The lymph nodes might be seen as a classroom, or perhaps as the war room. Macrophages and dendritic cells migrate to lymph nodes near the site of infection — or transplant — and display the foreign antigens they've acquired. This alerts T helper cells (Th cells), which release a variety of cytokines that direct the evolving immune response. CTLs spend most of their existence as T cytotoxic (Tc) cells. They're activated cytokines, interacting with antigens that are present in combination with MHC-I molecules.

Natural killer (NK) cells are T-cells with an attitude. They're usually among the first combative immune cells to arrive at the site of an infection, followed as much as a day or two later by CTLs. Both types of cells kill by releasing enzymes that literally eat holes through the membrane of infected or foreign cells.

When B cells are activated by antigens and cytokines in

the lymph nodes, they begin to manufacture antibodies in enormous quantities. Antibodies are wondrously efficient little molecules usually depicted in texts as looking like a capital "Y." The base of the Y attaches to the antigen on cell surfaces while the two arms reach away from the cell to attach to passing NK cells and macrophages that have been drawn to the area. The B cells are clonal, producing only one specific antibody. They do so with such efficiency that foreign cells are literally coated with these proteins. Cells coated with antibodies are like a spare rib painted with barbecue sauce and thrown to a pack of jackals: they don't stand a chance.

All these cells (Th, NK, and B) undergo clonal prolif-eration. This is an important point. Each NK cell induced to proliferate and attack foreign cells displaying a specific antigen is a clone, an exact copy of the parent NK cell. The result is millions of NK cells that are bent on the destruction of only those cells displaying the antigen. All others are spared.

The same holds true for Th cells and B cells. An ener-gized immune response is not a blind reaction. It doesn't rage through veins and arteries, attacking everything it encounters. These cells are trained to go only after cells that display one specific antigen.

After the offending virus, bacterium, or tissue has

been destroyed, the immune response quiets down. Most of the immune cells that led it die, but a few T and B cells remain to hold the memory of the specific antigen that sparked the response. This is the memory that confers immunity. The next time a pathogen appears, for example a measles bacterium, no antigen processing is necessary. The cells instantly recognize on the bacterial surface antigens they may have encountered years before and immediately destroy the germ before it has a chance to establish itself.

There is much that I have not explained about the immune system and its response to foreign tissue. The material presented here is little more than a sketch on a napkin. Texts on immunology depict the immune response by showing dendritic cells, macrophages, Th cells, NK cells, B cells, and swarms of antibodies circling a hapless invading cell like attackers around a wagon train. Arrows depicting the release of cytokines and the cells they affect swirl in all directions. Such a depiction, allegedly presented to clarify the immune response, makes a map of the New York City subway system seem simple by comparison.

It's this complexity, this subtle intricacy, that gives the immune system its power. Books have been written and research conducted by thousands of investigators for half a century or longer; new insights into aspects of the system appear in journals monthly; and still we don't completely understand the immune system.

But we're learning, and now we understand enough to intervene on behalf of our patients. Our knowledge of the immune system allows us to plan to prevent the system from attacking and destroying the different tissues that constitute the structure of the proposed face transplant. Each of these tissues displays it own antigens. Each of these antigens prompts a strong but subtly different immunological response from the transplant recipient. If it were not inhibited, the host's immune response to the different transplant tissues and their antigens would be massive. But it can be stopped with immunosuppressive therapy.

Dampening the recipient's immune response to prevent graft rejection also weakens the patient's response to the viral, bacterial, and fungal factors that we encounter on a daily basis. To reduce the threat of infection, we will supplement the immunosuppressive regimen with antibacterial and antiviral medications.

The regimen currently proposed for a face transplant recipient has been established in other composite-tissue allograft procedures. Although the regimen has been shown to work, it's a blunt instrument, an intervention that reduces the entire immune response. One thrust of research is to devise immunosuppressive agents that function with more precision that those we now have. These would be agents that suppress only the immune response to foreign tissue, while leaving intact the system's ability to respond to infection.

Some of this work is under way in my laboratory at Cleveland Clinic. The first experiments to test the power of immunosuppressive agents during rejection of composite tissue allografts were designed in my laboratory in Salt Lake City.

When my chairman, friend, and mentor Graham Lister retired, we moved to Cleveland Clinic, where I found great opportunity to continue my research on immunological challenges and responses which are unique to composite tissue allograft transplants. We are testing these challenges and responses by traveling several paths simultaneously. We're using antibodies to interfere with specific aspects of the immune response. We're also working on regimens that essentially fool the immune system into accepting transplanted tissue as its own.

One of the immune system's more powerful abilities is to manufacture antibodies that target a specific antigen, usually on the surface of a bacterium or virus. We have learned how to do the same thing in the laboratory. B cells produce antibodies in seconds. We need more time.

The goals of transplant research, what might be

considered the holy grail of the search, is to create an immunosuppressive therapy that will allow a recipient to accept a donor transplant as if it were his or her own and to eliminate altogether the need for chronic or lifelong immunosuppressive therapy. Current drugs create tolerance for transplanted tissue and organs at the cost of weakening the immune system's response to infectious organisms. The drugs are expensive and not without side effects. For the past several years, my laboratory colleagues and I have been looking for a way to leap over the MHC barrier. We have met with a degree of experimental success, as is demonstrated by the chimeras we have created.

What are chimeras? We borrowed the name from Greek mythology, which describes a beast of several parts, including the head of a lion, the body of a goat, and the tail of a snake. We have created several. They're not exactly as dramatic as their mythological counterparts. In fact, it would be difficult to tell one of our chimeric rats from a standard rat in the adjoining cage. That's exactly what we hoped for.

Our first efforts began with a standard dose of cyclosporin A (CsA) combined with alpha-beta T-cell antibody, which we gave to one breed of rats receiving hind-limb transplants from another. These breeds are normally incompatible, and the hind-limb transplant is a composite-tissue transplant containing several tissues, including bone and bone marrow. The drugs were administered at standard dosages begun shortly before the operation and tapered for 35 days, when treatment was stopped. The rats lived for more than two years, with no signs of rejection.

This success bred further research. We conducted a similar experiment, but this time the drug protocol lasted only seven days. We then conducted another experiment with CsA, but this time we used antilymphocyte serum rather than the antibody. Treatment was offered for 21 days and then stopped. Again the animals and their grafts survived long after cessation of therapy.

Analysis of blood and tissue showed that the recipient animals harbored chimeric cells. The rats were neither one breed nor another, but a combination of both. As such, the recipients tolerated the foreign tissue as if it were their own.

This is a start. It is a long, long way from a bench in a laboratory to a transplant patient's bedside, and there are many stumbling blocks along the path. But my colleagues and I in Cleveland and around the world share one characteristic: we are persistent.

෨෧

CHAPTER 9

The Ethical Considerations

BOTH CHANCE AND choice play a role in the selection of a candidate for a face transplant. Chance plays a role in all our lives. Chance led the young Finnish woodchopper to glance in the wrong direction as the ax fell. Chance allowed me to be on call the day he was brought into the ER. I knew chance would result in the disfigurement of the man or woman who would soon receive another's face.

That's where chance ends and choice begins. When I first proposed a face transplant procedure, I determined that the candidate would choose us, not the reverse. Doctors spend their professional lives working with people in need, and any good doctor soon learns how to persuade a patient of the necessity of a medical regimen or procedure. This is a virtue in most instances. Convincing a patient to quit smoking, follow a diet, or have a cancerous kidney removed is right and proper. Indeed, to do otherwise would be unethical.

However, convincing a person to submit to what is clearly defined as an experimental procedure would be unethical at best and the height of presumptive arrogance at worst. Neither I nor anyone on my team has sought patients for a face transplant, although through work and colleagues we all know of many potential candidates. Instead we've relied on the publicity the proposed procedure has received in the scientific, medical, and lay media to attract candidates. This has been successful. We have a number of candidates.

The candidates we have seen to date and those who will follow undergo evaluation by the most rigorous clinical and psychological examinations devised. Nothing is left to chance.

Our first transplant recipient was the first to successfully navigate an array of clinical and psychological screening procedures that have taken years to design. The effort involved me, every member of the transplant team, and Cleveland Clinic's Institutional Review Board (IRB).

THE DEPARTMENT OF Bioethics at Cleveland Clinic occupies a suite of new offices on the sixth floor of a recently completed structure bearing the singularly uninspired designation of *Building J.* It might be said that these important offices owe their existence to four events spread across more than two millennia of Western history: the misattribution of quote to a Greek philosopher, a German trial, a medical experiment conducted by the U.S. Public Health Service, and a medical article written by the son of a Kansas City night watchman.

The Latin phrase *Primum non nocere* is translated as "First, do no harm." Most people, including many medical professionals, assume that the phrase is or was part of the oath of medicine advanced by Hippocrates 24 centuries ago. But that specific Latin phrase is not in the medical oath (Hippocrates was Greek, for one thing). It may have been drawn from the book *Of the Epidemics*, in which Hippocrates wrote, "Declare the past, diagnose the present, foretell the future; practice these acts. As to diseases, make a habit of two things — to help, or at least to do no harm." The phrase rarely appeared in medical literature until the mid-1800s, when it began to show up in English and American medical articles and texts. Regardless of its origin, the concept is now one of the central tenets of modern medical ethics.

On December 9, 1946, presiding judge Walter B. Beals brought down his gavel with a definitive bang in the Palace of Justice in Nuremberg, Germany, and began the so-called "doctors' trial" of 23 Nazi physicians and program administrators. It ended nine months later. Five defendants were acquitted. Eleven were given prison terms ranging from ten years to life. Seven were sentenced to death.

During the nine-month trial the judges heard horrifying stories of human medical experimentation. This was a crime none had ever confronted. The justices sought input from Dr. Leo Alexander, a Tufts University psychiatrist who had spent days interviewing both the defendants and the subjects of their experiments. The doctor offered the justices a "memo" which the justices, in handing down their verdicts, expanded into ten cardinal points now known as the Nuremberg Code.

Medical ethics had been the sole preserve of the medical profession for millennia, and through the centuries, physicians for the most part held to strict codes. But laws, codes, and guidelines are made for the few who would violate them, not for the many who remain true to the profession. The wrenching descriptions of what humans could do to humans in the name of science showed the necessity for guidelines. More than 2,000 years after Hippocrates advised "First, do no harm," a strict set of guidelines governing human medical experimentation was now on paper.

In 1964, the Nuremberg Code was succeeded by the Declaration of Helsinki, a set of ethical principles governing human experimentation adopted by the World Medical Association. This document also established the principle of informed consent as central to ethics in research involving human subjects. The Helsinki document is distinguished in that it is perhaps the first instance in which the medical community sought to regulate itself rather than turn to governmental control.

Two years later, Dr. Henry K. Beecher, an anesthetist at the Harvard Medical School and the son of a Kansas City night watchman, published an article in the *New England Journal of Medicine* titled "Ethics and Clinical Research." The doctor identified 22 "unethical or questionably ethical studies" recently published in highly respected but unnamed medical journals. The article was a bomb dropped dead center into the nation's flourishing biological research effort.

The 22 articles were not isolated studies. Dr. Beecher reviewed 100 medical articles published consecutively in 1964 in respected journals and found that 12 of them raised serious ethical concerns. This endeavor implied that

10 percent of all U.S. research involving human subjects stood on shaky ethical foundations.

The article sparked a furor. Leading American physicians and academicians stated angrily that it was impossible for the U.S. medical establishment to conduct unethical medical experiments on humans in the light of the Nuremberg revelations only 20 years before. The debate continued until 1972, when an Associated Press article exposed the infamous Tuskegee Syphilis Experiment, so named for the Tuskegee Institute, the college that served as one of the centers for the study.

For forty years, between 1932 and 1972, the United States Public Health Service allowed diagnosed syphilis to proceed untreated in 399 African Americans without their knowledge. The health service said the purpose of the experiment was to compare the progress of the disease in African Americans to what was known about its progress in Caucasians. But there were no Caucasians in the study.

In response to the public outcry, in 1974, the U.S. Congress established the National Commission for the Protection of Human Subjects of Biomedical and Behavioral Research. In 1979, the commission published the Belmont Report, named for the Belmont Conference Center in Elkridge, Maryland, where the committee met and drafted the document.

The Belmont Report elaborates three principles: respect for the individual, beneficence, and justice. Respect for the individual is the concept that underlies informed consent. Such consent rests on two principles: No procedure, experimental or otherwise, should be performed on an individual without his or her consent, and it is the responsibility of the practitioner to ensure that the patient understands the procedure and all its possible consequences well enough to make a rational decision.

Beneficence involves balancing risks and benefits, perhaps one of the most challenging endeavors in experimental procedures. After all, these studies are called "experimental" precisely because the responses to the intervention, though anticipated, are not guaranteed and side effects may be completely unknown. Regardless of the procedure being considered or the study being designed, there must be clear indications that if successful, it will do some good. There's to be no more "Let's try this and see what happens." The days of conducting experiments simply to acquire knowledge that might or might not be practical are gone, and good riddance to them.

The final concept, justice, strikes at the remnants of the class system. For centuries the subjects of experimentation were drawn from the lower classes, from charity wards and prisons. The beneficiaries of the new procedures and medications that evolved from these experiments were invariably the upper classes. The lower classes received the medical rewards of their sacrifices only when those rewards became common and affordable. This was a despicable practice that needed to end if the principles of justice in medicine were to be achieved.

These events and the resultant laws, regulations, guidelines, and concepts occurred against a backdrop of sweeping social change.

Unquestioned acquiescence to a physician's decisions and directions survived 2,000 years of tumultuous history but didn't survive the civil rights movement, the women's rights movement, or the upheaval wrought by the Vietnam War. Prior to World War II, a doctor's authority was unquestioned. When in 1796, Edward Jenner dribbled secretions containing cowpox into lacerations he had made in the thin arm of young James Phipps, the boy's father no doubt stood by silently. The human experiment with the farm lad as preventive medicine today would have resulted in the doctor losing his license and probably bearing the costs and damages of a hefty lawsuit.

Patients are now autonomous; they are partners with physicians. The decisions they make regarding their treatment now carry a weight equivalent to the advice of the most highly trained and respected specialists in medicine.

The value and necessity for an institutional ethics department staffed with men and women trained to identify and resolve ethical issues is reflected in Cleveland Clinic's ethics department's growth. When the Cleveland Clinic ethics department was formed in 1983, it consisted of its chairman, Dr. George Kanoti, and one secretary. Today the Department of Bioethics houses eight ethicists and a fellow, each of whom has a specialty or special area of interest. The office also holds an eight-person research and support staff. The department focuses on issues directly affecting patients, physicians, and health care. The institution's ethics committee is a separate entity that confronts ethical issues on a far broader range of subjects.

The primary responsibility of the Department of Bioethics is to ensure that all the parties involved in making a medical decision base that decision on sound ethical principles: respect for the individual, beneficence, and justice. The department is there to provide not answers but the tools and directions to find them.

By one route or another, almost all ethical questions return to the central concept of informed consent. Because the candidate for a face transplant is essentially a full partner in determining the success of the procedure, it's the responsibility of all involved to ensure that the patient is both intellectually and psychologically fit. Intellectually the candidate must be as capable of assessing the complexities and challenges of the proposal as any of the specialists involved. The patient need not have a degree in biology, but must be intelligent enough to absorb and understand information about the procedure. All the preoperative, perioperative, and postoperative procedures, all the challenges and possible outcomes must be carefully laid out and explained. Regardless of the skill, experience, and stature of the medical personnel involved, it's still the patient who has to make the hard decision about whether the operation will proceed.

Finding patients who meet the intellectual criteria is not difficult. Many people have the capacity to understand the physical and biological aspects of a transplant. Ensuring that someone is psychologically fit to undergo the experience is another and perhaps more difficult endeavor. Clint Hallam, the Australian who received the first hand transplant in France and later had it removed at his own request, is an example of an error in judgment made in selecting a candidate for a transplant.

Dr. Katrina Bramstedt of the Clinic's bioethics staff specializes in transplant ethics and was a primary contributor to the ethical discussion that ensued when a face transplant was first proposed.

She notes that transplant recipients, in addition to bearing a responsibility toward themselves, also bear a responsibility to the donor for the organs or limbs they receive. Organ, tissue, and limb recipients must recognize that they are custodians of a rare and valuable resource. All transplant tissue is scarce, which means that when an organ is given to one individual, it's denied to another. The sacrifice made by a facial transplant donor is greater than that made by donors of internal organs, since he or she is denying family members the traditional support of an open-casket funeral, a last chance for loved ones to say goodbye to someone they recognize. Recipients have an expanded moral obligation to honor the donor's sacrifice.

The candidate for the procedure must also be able to assess risks and benefits free of prejudice. The candidate can be assumed to be inherently biased in favor of the procedure. Disfigurement and the desire to escape the social prison created by disfigurement are what bring the candidate to the institution as a volunteer. Most candidates aren't inquiring about the *possibility* of a new face — they *want* a normal face. Can such people be expected to balance risks and benefits impartially when the risks and benefits are currently imprecisely defined?

Another responsibility of the ethicist is to ensure that

the medical team proposing the procedure does not unduly influence the patient. The team members wouldn't have proposed the procedure if they weren't certain of success. The confidence demonstrated by the numerous specialists attending the candidate can bias the patient.

"What do you think I should do, Doctor?"

It's a question we hear every day. In this case, the response must be "That's a question you'll have to answer yourself." Doctors have opinions, often strong ones, and this isn't the way we like to answer questions from patients.

It should be said that not everyone shared the confidence of the team assembled at Cleveland Clinic. There are a number of institutions around the world whose staffs are fully capable of conducting a face transplant. But after weighing the risks and benefits, they have decided to wait. Waiting, however, also involves a cost. Waiting is a decision to deny someone a procedure that may benefit his or her life.

These are but a few of the ethical questions my team and I confronted when we first began to consider this procedure. These questions can be like Russian *matryoshka* dolls: Take one apart, and inside there is another. And inside that one, there is yet another. The job of the bioethicist is not to provide answers, but to make sure that the right paths are followed when answers are sought.

These paths will differ from nation to nation and from culture to culture. The issues we tackled and resolved at the Clinic and in this nation are also being met in Britain, France, Japan, China, and other countries. The answers aren't always the same. I believe the primary authority is a well-educated patient, one who knows the risks and can weigh them against a need for some degree of normalcy in a complex society. The decision belongs to the patient.

EVERY CLINIC, HOSPITAL, and health-care institution doing research of any nature has an IRB. This history that shaped informed consent is also the foundation of IRBs. But unlike the concept of consent, which evolved over time, IRBs have a birth date. They were created overnight with the publication of a short memo issued by the United States Public Health Service on February 8, 1966:

No new, renewal, or continuation research or research training grant in support of clinical research and investigation involving human beings shall be awarded by the Public Health Service unless the grantee has indicated in the application the manner in which the grantee institution will provide prior

> *review of the judgment of the principal investigator*
> *or program director by a committee of his institu-*
> *tional associates. This review should ensure an inde-*
> *pendent determination: (1) of the rights and welfare*
> *of the individual or individuals involved, (2) of*
> *the appropriateness of the methods used to secure*
> *informed consent, and (3) of the risks and potential*
> *medical benefits of the investigation. A description*
> *of the committee associates who will provide the*
> *review shall be included in the application.*

This simple policy memo brought massive changes in the structure of U.S. health-care institutions. Today, the IRB at Cleveland Clinic consists of 13 primary voting members: two hematologist/oncologists, two nursing specialists, a critical-care cardiologist, an orthopedic surgeon, a critical-care pediatrician, a pharmacist, a neuropsychologist, a radiologist, a social worker, a bioethicist, and an attorney. There is a reserve of 13 alternates who possess a similar range of experience and expertise. No clinical research on human subjects is conducted at the Clinic or anywhere else in the United States without IRB approval.

The guideline for the board's decision, the point where discussion begins and ends, is the research protocol. This is a document that spells out in exacting detail every aspect of the proposed procedure, from selecting a candidate and the details of the surgery to the follow-up immunotherapy and care after the tissue has been transplanted.

The protocol is notable for two reasons. It illustrates that the procedure under consideration involves more than a collection of highly trained medical specialists; it is being evaluated by an institution and some of the best minds that institution is able to bring together once a week in a conference room. Also, the protocol describes the clinical and psychological characteristics that we demand to see potential candidates demonstrate.

A protocol for a new surgical procedure, especially one that has never before been attempted, is an extensive document.

Presenting my protocol to the Clinic's institutional review board was much like defending my doctoral thesis, the difference being that the thesis presentation was over in an afternoon. Defending the transplant protocol took more than nine months.

WHEN I FIRST appeared before the IRB members on December 16, 2003, the board's offices were at the end of a long, dull corridor in the basement of an old stone building on Chester Avenue in Cleveland. I'd sent the office copies of the protocol much earlier to give the board members time to review it and frame questions. A researcher presenting a proposal to the board can gather some idea of how much interest the idea has generated by counting the number of coats on the rack outside the meeting room. When I arrived, the rack was buried.

The secretary greeted me and asked me to be seated while she informed the board's chairman, Dr. Alan Lichtin, that I was in the office. A few moments later the doctor opened the door to the boardroom and invited me in.

The light filtering through the basement windows fell on a long table and a room jammed with individuals representing nearly every aspect of a major modern clinical institution. They had questions.

"Who wrote the consent form?"

"Who's seen it? Who's reviewed it?

"What are the legal ramifications?"

"What is proposed to be the candidate's psych profile?"

"Why have the French decided not to follow this protocol?"

"What is the position of the working party in Great Britain, and why are they presently refusing permission for their physicians to attempt the procedure?"

"What research have you personally conducted?"

"How is your approach different?"

"Why do you feel you are better suited to conduct this procedure than surgeons in Great Britain or even in Louisville?"

"Why does it have to be donor facial tissue? Why not tissue from elsewhere on the patient's body?"

"Who's going to pay for this?"

That's just a sample of the questions that filled the first 15 minutes of what would be several such meetings. They served a purpose. Most of the questions were anticipated, but some weren't.

For instance, if one of the board members had not asked me how much tissue was needed, I wouldn't have undertaken research showing how much area the skin of the face actually covers. It's substantial, and finding enough flesh elsewhere on a patient's body to replace an entire face would be difficult. This is one of the reasons why the initial procedure is going to be limited to patients whose damage or disfigurement is limited primarily to the face. Should the allograft be rejected, we will have to acquire tissue from the patient's body, an endeavor that would be rendered impossible if the patient had suffered extensive burns.

In the end, I won approval. I was told that one of the reasons the board accepted my protocol was the respect, patience, and perseverance I had shown. Apparently, some IRB conversations with prominent researchers seeking approval for experiments have been rather contentious, with more than one researcher slamming the boardroom door upon leaving—behavior the board is unlikely to find endearing.

After IRB approval, my next challenge was dealing with the media. I don't always look forward to encounters with the media, but I don't shy away from them either. It's my responsibility, as it is the responsibility of all doctors and scientists, to present information, new ideas, and advances to our own medical community and to the public through the media. In modern democracies, science advances only with the acceptance and support of the public it serves. Patient advocates, institutional review boards, informed-consent forms and formulas, ethical and legal constraints, and a host of other medical services were created to serve the public and the patient, not the doctor or science.

I met the media on occasion during conferences and conventions. The reporters were usually specialists developing articles for specialty medical publications. These articles seldom reached beyond their target audience of physicians and research scientists.

My concern for the facial transplant procedure I was

advocating was that it carried the potential to be overly dramatized. If information were mishandled or if the procedure were misrepresented, it would be all too easy to unleash what is called "the Frankenstein syndrome." The press might focus on the dramatic cosmetic changes rather than the social, psychological, and health problems that would be resolved. (After the IRB approval was announced I was contacted by some people from Hollywood wanting to know whether I'd be interested in serving as an advisor in the making of *Face Off II*, a sequel to the film in which John Travolta and Nicolas Cage traded faces. I wasn't.)

When it seemed that Cleveland Clinic's institutional review board was moving toward approval of the face transplant, it became clear that both the Clinic and I would be drawing the attention of most of the major news enterprises — large and small newspapers, magazines, and radio and television networks. I turned to Eileen Sheil, executive director of the Clinic's public and media relations department. It's her job to anticipate telephone queries from major news outlets before those callers know they'll be making them.

She and I devised a strategy for meeting what we both suspected would be a media onslaught. Harlan Spector of Cleveland's *The Plain Dealer* had written frequently on medical issues. He'd be given a complete background on the proposed procedure, including a history of transplants, the rationale behind the proposal, ethical issues involved, the way the procedure would be conducted, and my biography. Spector was given this information with the understanding that the story wouldn't be published until the IRB announced its approval. And though approval seemed likely, it was by no means guaranteed.

Our strategy was not to play favorites or to give a local reporter an advantage, but to create a foundation article for the other media representatives who'd be calling. Many of the reporters seeking information and interviews would be unfamiliar with the science, medicine, and ethics of the procedure. We'd be able to tell them, "Our local paper has a pretty good article on the subject. Give it a quick read and call back." When they did, they could ask specific questions rather than seek an entire medical education.

There was another reason we wanted the media to publish the most accurate information possible. We recognized that the story would draw a substantial amount of interest from potential candidates for the procedure. It was essential that innovative aspects of the procedure and its attendant risks be clearly stated. We didn't wish to raise false hopes, and conversely, we didn't want to discourage those who might become candidates.

On the whole, I'd say that the strategy worked. For me, it was a novel experience. For the Clinic's public relations department, it was just another long week.

CHAPTER 10

The Candidate

ALTHOUGH ANY NUMBER of people have tried to establish rules and measures for beauty and ugliness, they've invariably failed. Beauty truly is in the eye of the beholder. Beauty in one culture does not necessarily translate to beauty in the next, nor does beauty in one era become beauty in the next. A ghostly pale face in the 18th century was envied because it reflected a person of status, a member of the wealthy class who didn't spend his days laboring in the fields. Today it's the image of an individual who perhaps spends too much time in a cubicle. People of status have tans.

A search of the sociological, psychological, and scientific literature reveals how a face is perceived. Those with attractive features see their self-opinion validated in the smiles of passersby, the courtesy of store clerks, and even an occasional wink from someone of the opposite sex. The disfigured see quite a different reflection. They see startled and frightened looks, stares of disbelief, and gazes averted as oncoming strangers step aside and hurry past.

Philip Zimbardo, in his 1981 book *Shyness*, quotes a woman disfigured by an operation that removed a brain tumor: "I kept thinking, 'Why did this have to happen to me?'...I tried walking around my block, but I simply could not stand the mocking laughter of children, or the giggles of some neighbors. When I walked into the shops alone, clerks gave me disdainful glances, and occasionally would toss my purchases at me." Ultimately the jeers and sarcastic comments she encountered left the woman unwilling to leave her home. She remained a recluse for months.

Dr. Frances Cooke Macgregor of the Institute of Reconstructive Plastic Surgery at the New York University Langone Medical Center was a pioneer in studying the impact of disfigurement. In 1990 she wrote this observation about the many disfigured persons she had known: "In their attempts to go about their daily lives, people [with disfigurements] are subjected to visual and verbal assaults, and a level of familiarity from strangers not otherwise dared: naked stares, startled reactions, 'double takes,' whispering, remarks, furtive looks, curiosity, personal questions, advice, laughter, ridicule, and outright avoidance. Whatever form the behaviors may take, they generate feelings of shame, impotence, anger, and humiliation in their victims."

The impact of disfigurement is amplified by our society's continuing quest for youth and beauty, a quest whose roots disappear into the mists of history. No era is established as humanity's first attempts to enhance appearance, but such endeavors began before 3100 BC, the date established for the urns of unguents and cosmetic substances unearthed by archaeologists in Egypt. The use of cosmetics to enhance beauty moved through the empires as they rose and fell — through Egypt, Greece, Rome, the medieval courts of Europe, and into today's Western civilization, in which cosmetics constitute an industry worth more than $200 billion a year.

It would be a disservice to those who are disfigured to spend much time discussing Western culture's obsession with youth and beauty. Our faces are more than visages to be adorned or veiled. They are essential to our communication with the world. It has been estimated that verbal communication conveys only 35 percent of the meaning we're expressing. Our looks, gestures, and body language carry 65 percent of the information received by the person at the other end of the conversation.

Dr. Paul Ekman, a retired professor of psychology at the University of California, San Francisco, is one of the pioneers of the study of facial expression and nonverbal communication. After studying the expression of emotions in cultures around the world, he said, "We found high agreement across members of diverse Western and Eastern literate cultures in selecting emotional terms that fit facial expression. We found evidence of universality in the spontaneous expressions and in expressions that were deliberately posed." It appears that facial expressions depicting specific emotions such as anger, joy, and disgust are not linked to a society or culture, but are part of our heritage as a species.

Dr. Ekman was not the first to advance the idea that facial expressions are universal and perhaps involuntary. In 1872, Charles Darwin published *The Expression of the Emotions in Man and Animals*. In an introduction to the reissue of Darwin's book, Dr. Ekman wrote: "His book is also a compendium of fascinating observations about the expressions of humans and other animals. We purse our lips when we concentrate on doing something, such as threading a needle. We open our mouth when listening intently. We want to touch with our faces those we love. We can bite affectionately, as do other animals. And so on, almost endlessly."

Imagine for a moment being able to do none of those things. Now you're beginning to grasp something of the burden a disfigured person.

Communication is a two-way street, a reality that increases the already substantial strain on disfigured people, who may avoid mirrors but can never avoid the way their disfigurement is reflected in the faces of others.

"The primary challenge encountered by individuals with facial disfigurement is the social response of the non-disfigured," wrote Thomas Pruzinsky, a professor at the Institute of Reconstructive Plastic Surgery at the New York University Langone Medical Center, about the challenges confronting individuals with facial disfigurement.

Changing Faces is a British organization that helps people with facial disfigurement cope with the challenges of everyday life. Dr. James Partridge, who was burned horribly in a car fire when he was 18 years old, founded it in 1992.

In his writings, Dr. Partridge lists the feelings and behaviors of disfigured people as well as the feelings and behaviors of those they encounter with the acronym SCARED. Disfigured persons feel *Self-conscious, Conspicuous, Angry* or *Anxious, Rejected, Embarrassed,* and *Different.* Their behavior is *Shy, Cowardly, Aggressive, Retreating, Evasive,* and *Defensive.*

Those whom they meet are also scared, according to Dr. Partridge. They feel *Shocked* or *Sorry, Curious* or *Confused, Anxious, Repelled, Embarrassed,* and *Distressed.* Their reactions include *Staring or Speechlessness, Clumsiness, Asking* or *Awkwardness, Rudeness or Recoiling,* and *Distractedness.*

The acronym might seem awkward, but it does suggest the complexity and range of human interactions that occur between unaffected persons and individuals with disfigurements. And it reflects the fact that all the emotions and feelings that rise in the observer and the observed are negative.

Others have studied this phenomenon. One scientist made careful observations of the response of the general public to the disfigured and reported that people generally stand farther away from those who are disfigured. During a typical encounter, they will also stand on the nondisfigured side of the individual. Members of the general public were seen to avoid the disfigured by increasing their pace, averting their gaze, and attempting to ignore the disfigured person's presence. They also tended to avoid looking directly at the facial anomaly, thus depriving the individual of an important aspect of communication.

Several psychologists have described the "hide-and-seek" behavior of the disfigured. They isolate themselves to avoid rejection while at the same time desperately wanting to be part of the crowd.

"Facial disfigurement and deformity are common causes of human suffering, much more common than a walk down the high street would suggest, as many afflicted will choose to hide from public gaze," wrote Dr. Duncan McGrouther, a professor of plastic surgery at the Royal Free and University College London Medical School, in the *British Medical Journal*.

These encounters with society can wound the psyche deeply. Those who are disfigured see themselves as others see them and bury their emotions in their gut. It's hard to grasp from the scientific literature any idea of the percentage of the disfigured who are psychologically damaged by their disease. It appears that there has been no definitive study of the problem, although it can be assumed to be common. How common? A few studies have been conducted that offer some clues.

One 2004 study from a hospital in Dublin, Ireland, suggests that psychiatric problems could be widespread. The hospital's plastic surgeons assessed the psychological health of patients referred for plastic surgery during the year 2001. They reported, "The majority of patients had significant existing psychiatric illness, had made a suicide/parasuicide attempt, or were burn patients."

At the University of Oslo in Norway, psychiatric follow-up of 70 burned adults conducted between 3 and 13 years after their injuries found that 23 percent suffered from definite psychosocial problems. Patients whose injuries were more severe had problems more often (44 percent) than patients with minor injuries (16 percent) did.

The Oslo study is one of the few to associate extent of injury with incidence of psychiatric disturbance. Several studies have stated that the incidence of psychological problems is related not so much to the severity of the injury as it is to preexisting problems and the strength (or weakness) of the patient's support network, including relationships with family and friends.

Men, women, and children are horribly disfigured by congenital deformities, accidents, and necessary medical procedures such as surgery to remove malignant tissue. Many of the procedures used to correct these insults still employ the principle of removing a patch of flesh from an unobtrusive location on a person's body and transplanting it to the face. There are patients today who, with courage, determination, and forbearance, undergo 20, 30, and 40 or more such procedures in an effort to restore their appearance to a socially acceptable state.

Society has, to say the least, granted social acceptance to cosmetic procedures. They're now the stuff of television drama and reality shows. It's impossible to count the number of brow lifts, eyelid procedures, neck tucks, liposuctions, lip enhancements, and facelifts conducted annually in the United States and around the world. The great majority of these surgeries are conducted in the name of beauty — or vanity, to put it more critically.

However, there remains hesitancy, even controversy, when the subject of a total face transplant is raised. It's true that the procedure is far more complex than many of the cosmetic jobs now considered routine. But the procedure is possible, as has been demonstrated in both the laboratory and the operating room. It's odd that society should approve of so many procedures that do no more than enhance an individual's otherwise acceptable features, yet be critical of a procedure that will allow disfigured people to reenter a world that has cast them into seclusion.

WE BELIEVED THAT the first candidate would likely be a burn patient whose damage did not significantly affect the underlying musculature that controls movement and expression. The candidate might have a functional impairment such as an inability to close his or her eyes or mouth, handicaps not uncommon in faces badly scarred by burns and restoration attempts. Patients with missing noses, lips, and eyelids have not been excluded from consideration. Restoring dynamic facial functions would make the success of the procedure all the more rewarding. Another requirement of the IRB clinical protocol is that candidates for the transplant must have exhausted all other possible therapies to correct function and disfigurement.

Patients with a history of cancer, diabetes, or certain infections are ineligible. After the transplant, the candidate will be placed on a regimen of potent immunosuppressive drugs. These agents will prevent the immune system from attacking the transplant; they'll also weaken the system's response to a range of diseases that includes cancer and diabetes. Although these diseases may never become a threat, we're taking no chances. Our intention is to do everything possible to stack the odds in favor of success.

Determining who is clinically eligible for the procedure is simpler than determining who is psychologically eligible. A patient's clinical status is composed of characteristics that can be seen and measured, but a person's psychological profile doesn't register in terms of white blood cell counts or electrocardiograms. Surgeons can palpate the scars that lie across a young woman's face and derive an idea of how deep they go, but when it comes to palpating psychological scars or even finding them, another type of expertise is needed.

Dr. Scott S. Meit, vice chairman of psychology at the Clinic, assembled the psychological profile for transplant candidates and became a central specialist in screening potential candidates for the procedure. Dr. Meit was recruited to Cleveland from the University of West Virginia in Morgantown in 2005. Upon his arrival, Dr. Meit found a pile of responsibilities lying on his desk, one of which was to draw the psychological profile of a candidate most likely to contribute to the success of the face transplant procedure. The second was to help identify that candidate.

Although the procedure is new and unique, defining eligibility criteria was not as difficult as might be thought. Dr. Meit's first job was to identify individuals capable of providing informed consent. He had any number of tools and instruments for evaluating an individual's ability to understand, analyze, evaluate, and respond to proposals for clinical procedures.

The phrase *tools and instruments* is a wonderful bit of medical terminology that conjures up the image of a psychiatrist poking around under a patient's skull the way a mechanic might root around the engine compartment of a cranky Ford. Yet the phrase actually refers to validated questionnaires that can be administered easily and that provide reliable results.

The initial interviews and testing identifies candidates who are intelligent enough to understand the general principles of the procedure, the nature of the benefits, the degree of risk, the consequences of failure, and the responsibilities inherent in a lifelong regimen of immunosuppression.

Other qualities sought by Dr. Meit and the transplant team are tougher to identify. These include psychological stability, resiliency, responsibility, and self-reliance.

One of the more important questions involved in assessing stability is the presence or absence of depression. It'd be easy to assume that anyone bearing the weight of a horribly disfigured face would harbor some degree of depression, but that's not necessarily so. People don't necessarily respond to traumatic events, ill health, handicaps, or disfigurement with depression, although depression can be present. The problem is that self-neglect and absent-mindedness are among its symptoms. These characteristics and others associated with depression cannot be tolerated in a person who is going to be required to follow a strict lifelong regimen of immunosuppressive drugs.

Accident survivors can have other psychological impairments. Two of the more common are post-traumatic stress disorder and survivor guilt. These closely related but separate disorders stem from traumatic events that may or may not leave physical scars but do leave psychological ones. They share many of the same symptoms, including emotional numbness, sleep disturbances, depression, anxiety, irritability, explosive anger, and a feeling of guilt for having survived events that may have taken the lives of companions or loved ones. These disorders and their symptoms are challenging to treat, and patients experiencing them can show wide variability in their responses to therapy, making them unlikely candidates for the face transplant.

Resiliency is the ability to cope, to bob and weave. The term is somewhat synonymous with the psychological term *ego strength*. Ego is said to be the component of the psyche that gives us personality, our way of dealing with both the external world of societal rules and demands and the internal world of desire and need. Ego strength is defined as the possession of a certain self-knowledge and objectivity in understanding the world and its ways. Ego strength also embodies the ability to plan or organize activities across periods ranging from hours to years, along with the ability to choose those alternatives that will lead to designated goals.

Psychological responsibility involves understanding that personal actions have consequences, that a path through life can be plotted and followed, while at the same time recognizing that unexpected events can and do disrupt life plans. A 22-question instrument known as the Achterberg and Lawlis Health Attribution Test allows specialists like Dr. Meit to assess the way individuals apportion responsibility for their lives and health. The responses to the test's questions are weighted and cast into three categories: "internal," "chance," and "powerful others."

A person who assigns his fate to internal variables is a person who takes responsibility for his actions and circumstances. Such a person not only believes he can do something about improving his health, but will do so.

Someone who assigns aches, pains, and handicaps to chance, fate, or bad luck may adopt a "why bother?" attitude toward therapy.

The "powerful others" category encompasses people who feel their lives are charted by parents, bosses, politicians, and shadowy political forces. As far as their health is concerned, such individuals would put nurses, doctors, and hospitals in the role of powerful others whom they allow to run their lives.

The answers to the 22 questions can be displayed as a three-slice pie chart. For patients undergoing medical procedures that involve extensive follow-up therapy or rehabilitation, specialists like it when the "internal" slice of the pie is fat.

A candidate should also be self-reliant or independent. This is a description not of a loner but of someone who is comfortable as an individual in a circle of friends and family. It's someone who is neither too humble nor too arrogant to ask for help and support when it's needed. And the support should be there. Having a strong friends-and-family support network favors the candidate and bodes well for the success of the procedure.

CHAPTER 11

When the Time Comes

I'VE BEEN PRACTICING medicine for more than 30 years. I didn't begin my career with the aim of conducting a face transplant, but I started to move in that direction when I treated the hands of burn victims. Since turning toward that goal, I haven't swerved.

I knew that, at some unpredictable hour of some unpredictable day, the telephone would ring and the voice at the other end of the line would say that she has spoken with the family of a deceased patient who has signed a donor card, and that the family has given the transplant coordinator full formal consent. The paperwork is complete. All forms have been signed and witnessed.

In addition to donating internal organs, the donor will offer a face to another.

This call will not initiate the transplant procedure. Another call has to be made to a candidate to determine availability and state of health. If the candidate has a cold, the flu, or any other infection, or is taking medications for such illnesses, the procedure is off; the candidate's immune system is already active and occupied. Remember, the transplant procedure requires that the recipient's immune system be modulated. The system will by no means be shut down, but it will be turned down. This can't be done in patients who need their immune systems to fight infection.

The recipient must also be available, which means being no more than a certain number of hours away from Cleveland Clinic. Practice with cadavers has given a reasonably accurate idea of how long the procedure will take, from the time preparations begin on the donor to the time the recipient is wheeled from the OR into the postanesthetic care unit. But one critical factor is unknown: the length of time required to get to the donor's location and back with the transplanted tissue. If the donor is already in the Clinic, it may take only minutes. If the donor is in one of the many participating institutions around the Midwest, it may take hours.

The tissues to be transplanted can be kept viable for up to ten hours, another factor in the equation. The candidate has to be able to get to the Clinic in time to undergo several hours of preparation. If that can't be done within what is now an unknown time period, the procedure will have to be canceled. Then we wait for another call.

If the patient is healthy and available, a cascade of calls will be made to alert medical professionals and everyone else associated with the procedure that the first step leading to a full face transplant has been taken. No questions will need to be asked. The protocols have been long established. Every aspect of the now rapidly evolving procedure has been carefully planned. All participants know where to go and what to do when they get there.

There will be two teams of three to four surgeons each. One team will retrieve the allograft from the donor. The second will prepare the patient to receive a new face.

A third team, one not integral to the face transplant itself, will be at the donor's institution to recover organs. We anticipate that the donor will be offering more than facial tissue. The people who sign those small donor cards tucked in their wallets or purses harbor a philosophy borne of an astounding courage and generosity, and a profound sense of obligation to their fellow human beings.

This generosity seldom has limits. Few organ donors offer only their hearts or only their lungs or only their kidneys. The message they're communicating is *Everything I have has served me well. Now it's yours. Use it with love and to enhance the lives of others.*

There won't be a great flurry of activity with doctors striding through halls shouting orders and nurses rushing to grab instruments. This won't be a televised hospital drama that comes to a conclusion in an hour. Indeed, for many of those involved, one of the procedure's most difficult aspects will be the waiting. There will be a lot of that.

Nurses will start moving long before the surgeons begin to gather. Operating rooms need to be scheduled — not a minor point. The ORs need to be large. Each room will have to accommodate a team of three or more surgeons, all of whom will be accompanied by assistants.

Modern hospitals are tight ships and costly to run. Once the lights go on in an OR, a budgetary clock starts ticking. Because operating rooms are expensive, they are seldom left standing vacant; procedures are scheduled weeks, sometimes months, in advance. When the transplant procedure is initiated, the donor's OR will be occupied for four to six hours. The recipient's OR may be needed for 12 hours or longer. This means that there's more to preparing an OR than opening the door and turning on the lights. Doctors and patients who have scheduled elective (nonemergency) procedures will have to be notified of schedule changes.

Technicians will run dozens of tests on the mechanical devices that are now essential and common in every modern OR to ensure that they are functioning properly and producing accurate readings. Scrub nurses (a terrible name, by the way, for essential, highly trained medical professionals) will begin preparing and laying out the instrumentation, sutures, and dressings that they know will be needed.

The first clinical actions to be taken will be to acquire a complete serology and tissue typing of the donor's tissues to ensure that they're compatible with those of the recipient. This analysis may take several hours. It's not conducted solely for the benefit of the face allograft recipient; it's also crucial for the other patients who may be eligible to receive organs from the donor. During this time, the brain-dead donor will be on support systems that keep blood, nutrients, and oxygen flowing to vital organs and tissues. When it's been confirmed that serology and tissues are a match, all those involved will be contacted and told that the procedure is a go and that the first necessary steps have been taken. They'll be asked to go to their posts.

The Clinic's transplant coordinator will pick up a phone and, in a voice made confident and calm from having made many such calls, will inform the recipient that the donor tissues appear to be compatible with the patient's own.

The recipient will be met at the Clinic by the coordinator and an admissions nurse who will review the paperwork. Even though the procedure has been planned for months and years already, there will still be paperwork and forms to be signed. If the patient is accompanied by family and relatives, the coordinator will join them to explain the procedure as it unfolds, familiarize them with the hospital and its amenities, and help them through what will be long hours of watching bad television, pretending to read old magazines, and drinking too much coffee.

A transport nurse will take the recipient to the preoperative holding area, where a nurse will review the patient's charts to ensure completeness and administer preoperative medications. The anesthesiologist will join the nurse and recipient to explain how the anesthetics will be administered and what to expect from them.

It will be a piece of good luck if the donor is already in Cleveland Clinic. If that's the case, the operating rooms may be separated by only a few yards of hallway or even just a wall with a connecting door. But it's more likely that the donor will be in one of the many hospitals in northern Ohio or elsewhere in the Midwest that have agreed to participate in the effort. We'll have to drive or fly to the institution where the donor waits. Time is of the essence. We need not only to get to the donor's location but also to get back to the waiting recipient.

I'll travel with that first team. Although I developed the protocol for the procedure, conducted the essential research, argued its necessity, explained it to innumerable colleagues and critics and television show hosts, shepherded the proposal through the IRB, and trained for most of my life for what is to take place during the next several hours, I doubt that I will touch a scalpel. I will supervise. I have to make sure that when the donor tissue is removed, all vessels, nerves, and anatomical landmarks are photographed and identified. I have to be completely familiar with every minute aspect of the donor's face. If I'm directly involved, if I'm dissecting vessels on one side of the donor's face, I may lose a necessary familiarity with the character and location of vessels and nerves on the other side.

In preparing for the transplant, my colleagues and I conducted mock procedures on cadavers. Even when we were working in a bloodless field and the passage of time was no consideration, small errors crept in as they do in any complicated procedure.

For example, a surgeon concentrating on freeing a portion of the flap steps back to study his work before moving on and forgets to take a picture of the region. Photographs are our backup. They serve as reference points should we need them. They're a map of the battlefield.

With such a big undertaking, someone must serve as general, someone in a position to survey the entire landscape and monitor the actions of everyone involved. I can make the overall procedure more efficient if I'm free to move around the working surgeons, answering questions and offering guidance.

I'll be in constant contact with the recipient team in order to monitor the status of the recipient, to ensure that all required personnel are present and that the appropriate immunosuppressive drugs are on hand and ready to be administered, and to supervise a multitude of other details. I'll probably be a pain in the neck. It's part of my job.

Although brain-dead, the donor will be on support and breathing through a tracheostomy tube inserted into the windpipe through an incision in the neck. In all other transplant procedures oxygenated air is provided through a face mask, but in this instance the tube is required to allow unimpeded access to the donor's face. Heparin, a blood thinner, will be administered to suffuse the heart, the other organs, and the head to prevent blood clots from forming at the ends of vessels when they are severed. Once it's certain that the heparin has coursed through the donor's vasculature, the face transplant acquisition team will step away to let other surgeons acquire organs such as the heart and kidneys.

Work on the recipient will begin about 90 minutes before the anticipated arrival in the operating room of the recovered facial tissue. This requires careful calculation. The donor's surgical team has a good idea of how long it will take to remove the tissue, but there's also the issue of transport. If the donor is at the Clinic, work on the recipient will begin about 90 minutes before the donor procedure is complete. If the donor is in an institution remote from the Clinic, perhaps several hours' drive or flight by helicopter or plane, this transport time has to be considered as a factor in preparing the recipient.

One of the measures the recipient team will undertake while waiting is to identify and outline areas on the patient's body where skin can be recovered if the transplanted tissue should be rejected after the surgery.

This is another criterion for accepting candidates

into this transplant program. They must have large areas of undamaged skin available for recovery in the event of rejection. With advances in serology and tissue-typing during the last several decades and our more recent ability to manipulate the immune system, rejection is unlikely. But it remains a possibility. We have to be prepared for everything.

Fortunately facial tissue is less susceptible to ischemia, when cells are deprived of oxygen, than are organs such as the heart or lungs. Ischemia doesn't cause immediate cell death. Cells continue to function on stored energy reserves. This process of breaking down nutrients and using the energy is called metabolism. If metabolism stops, the cell dies.

All surgeons, regardless of their specialty or the organ and tissues they're working on, know how long a specific organ will last without blood. This knowledge is essential in many procedures. For instance, some kidney operations require that the major vessels serving the organ be clamped to minimize the loss of blood by the patient and to allow the surgeon to work in a blood-free environment. From the minute those vessels are clamped, the surgeon knows exactly how long he has to complete the procedure before cells in the organ begin to die.

Metabolism in an organ can't be stopped, but cooling

to a few degrees above freezing can slow metabolism and prolong organ viability. Freezing is out of the question. In 1987 a group of researchers at the University of Wisconsin created the biological equivalent of antifreeze. They called the fluid the "Wisconsin solution." This solution is composed of a variety of chemicals and nutrients that limit or prevent the cellular damage that would be caused by dramatic reductions in temperature.

This solution, cooled to 39.2 degrees Fahrenheit and suffused through an organ, slows metabolism to a near standstill but keeps the spark of life burning. It's fortunate for my specialty that under these conditions skin can remain vital for 10 to 12 hours. Muscle survives only half that time, about 6 hours. Thus we surgeons have a cushion, one that allows us to accept donor tissue located a significant distance from the recipient.

At some point during the day or evening, I'll call the recipient team and tell them that we anticipate walking into their OR with the donor tissue in about an hour and a half. Almost immediately after that call is made, the anesthesiologist will turn to the recipient and say, "It's time."

Like the donor, the recipient undergoes a tracheostomy to allow anesthesia to be administered. The reason is the same. The tracheostomy allows surgeons unimpeded access to the recipient's face. It will take 30 to 40 minutes to complete the tracheostomy and administer the anesthesia. Incisions will be made on both sides of the neck to give the surgeons access to the carotid arteries and jugular veins, the major vessels carrying blood to and from the face.

The next step is to wait for the arrival of the donor tissue. The surgeons may study the defects in the patient's face and even mark it to show where eventual incisions will be made. They'll review the procedure over and over again, the way a downhill skier imagines every turn and pitch of his course down the mountain before he enters the starting gate.

The actual transplant procedure will begin with the arrival of the donor tissue. The patient's carotids and jugulars will be clamped; the donor's tissue will be joined to these veins and arteries, and the clamps on the blood vessels will be opened. This should be a significant moment as dozens of eyes watch as the donor's skin begins to pink up. Any areas of white or blue will indicate an interruption of blood flow through the tissue and will have to be dealt with. It will also tell us of the effectiveness of the immunosuppressive agents given to the recipient before the procedure began. If there is to be a hyperacute rejection (an antibody-mediated rejection), it will begin the moment the clamps are released and blood begins flowing into the tissue.

When it has been shown that the transplant is viable and that the recipient's body is accepting it, the long, delicate labor of fixing the new tissue to old will begin.

The recipient's face will be removed. Although a substantial portion of the facial surface may be taken, the extent to which underlying structures such as muscles and bones will be included will be based on the extent of the patient's disfigurement. One of the early criteria in selecting a recipient was that the damage, though perhaps extensive, must be confined to the surface. However, after interviewing many patients with severe deformities where all facial structures and components were damaged, we concluded that despite challenges we have to consider transplanting muscles, bones, and specialized units such as nose, ears, eyelids, and lips in order to restore function and the appearance of the transplant patient.

Like the donor, the recipient's vessels and nerves will be incised carefully to preserve hemostasis (stoppage of blood flow), prevent clotting, and reduce risk of inflammation. Nerves will be the first structures to be joined because they usually lie deepest in tissue. The suturing of arteries and veins will follow. Depending on the damage to the recipient's face and its underlying tissue, sutures will be placed at various points in the donor tissue and tacked to facial ligaments in the recipient to prevent the tissue from sloughing off during the initial phases of healing. All this is exacting labor, demanding perhaps a touch of art. Many of the surgeons will be wearing jewelers' loupes. A surgical microscope will be in the OR and is likely to be used more than once during the procedure.

I've described the surgical aspects of the transplant procedure in a handful of paragraphs that you've read in a few minutes. All that has been described as well as much that hasn't will take place over 12 to 16 hours. It will seem like an excruciatingly long time, especially for the patient's family and friends, and I suspect that at certain moments during the procedure, one or more of the surgeons involved will be thinking the same thing. But I'll bet that once everything is completed, everyone involved will feel as if the time flew past.

At this point, the patient will be tied to innumerable monitoring devices that will be providing information on blood pressure, heart rate, the viability of the transplanted tissue, the flow of blood into and out of the tissue, the response of the recipient to the new tissue, and the response of the new tissue to the recipient. Intravenous lines will be funneling nutrients and drugs into the patient's system.

Among these will be analgesics to block pain, antiviral and antibacterial drugs, anticoagulants, and immunosuppressive agents.

The recipient will be wheeled to the postanesthetic care unit (or PACU, called the "pack-you" by everyone in the hospital) and upon arising from a deep anesthetic slumber will meet family and world with a new face. We'll know whether the procedure has been successful within 24 to 72 hours. Within this time frame, the patient will have come out of anesthesia. Blood flow into and out of the graft will be total and stable, and there will be no evidence of hyperacute rejection. Dressings will be put on and, as you might imagine, the patient will resemble a mummy. Given the extent of the procedure, substantial swelling is to be expected. A transport nurse will take the patient from PACU to the intensive care unit (ICU), where monitoring will continue for five days to a week.

The dressings will leave portions of the grafted tissue exposed to permit the "refill test." You can try this at home. Press your finger gently but firmly on the back of your hand for a few seconds. When you lift your finger, there will be a small white spot that will quickly regain color. If that spot had turned somewhat blue and remained so, it would indicate a venous problem: blood is not being carried away from the area. If the spot remains white or is slow to return to pink, it could indicate an arterial problem. There's a certain irony in the test, which the ICU nurses will administer frequently: with all the sophisticated devices and technological machinery available in a modern hospital, one of the most important and valuable tests we have for determining the success of a transplant is a nurse's touch.

From ICU, the patient will go to a post-op care ward for another ten days or so and then to a care unit, either in the hospital or nearby. I estimate that the return home will take place four to six weeks after surgery. During this recovery period medical and psychological counseling will be provided. A patient advocate will make sure that the recipient gets any care needed and provide advice on how to deal with family, friends, and the work environment.

A specialist will provide guidance on how to deal with the media. Of course the hospital will protect the patient's anonymity. But it's possible that the media will discover the identity of the transplant recipient. Imagine coming home to find that your disfigured neighbor has a new face. How could you (or anyone) possibly keep a secret like that from your family or the gang around the water cooler?

The patient will be monitored monthly for six months, then every other month or every three months for a year or longer, and then at regular intervals established between the patient and caregiver — for life.

It will be done. And for the patient and me, the reward will be something we're both waiting to see. A smile.

EPILOGUE

ONE LATE EVENING in early December 2008, I settled into bed to read my book before going to sleep. Suddenly my beeper and telephone began to ring. It was unusual to hear both ring simultaneously, and I had a strange feeling that the moment had arrived. I don't know why, but I hesitated for a moment before picking up the phone, as if I wanted to buy more time. I was hopeful and uncertain at the same time. Would the years of careful preparation and planning pay off? Were we truly ready? Would we change someone's life in the next 24 hours?

Finally, I picked up the phone and I heard a familiar voice on the other end of the line. It was the donation specialist. She said that she had spoken with a potential donor's family. She had explained the special request for a face donation, and the family had given full formal consent.

At that moment, I knew that the clock had started

running. We would have only a matter of time to organize the team, bring the patient to the hospital, notify her family, the ICU, and pharmacy, and book two side-by-side operating rooms with the required equipment, including instruments, microscopes, saws, and more.

In the back of my mind I knew that our transplant candidate had been waiting for this moment for a very long time. She needed the face transplant due to trauma that led to significant loss of her facial functions. She was not able to breathe, smell, or smile.

I was finally faced with the ability to proceed and follow the protocol we implemented four years earlier. I immediately called the team members.

It was close to midnight when I began calling all of the people on the list: the surgical team members, transplant coordinators, nurses, and most importantly, the patient. Even though it was getting late, every single person answered the phone and, without any hesitation, was ready to proceed.

THE FIRST NEAR-TOTAL U.S. face transplantation procedure began late in the afternoon hours of the next day and was completed 22 hours later. The procedure took place at Cleveland Clinic, and was completed by a team of 8 surgeons, 4 anesthesiologists, more than 20 nurses, and countless other technicians and assistants. This was a big undertaking and involved two fully staffed operating rooms going simultaneously.

As planned, my main job as the leader of the team was to ensure that everything went smoothly. At times this meant that I was scrubbed in on the donor recovery. At other times I was working with the microsurgical team on the anastomosis of the vessels. The years of research and preparation were not lost. The 22 hours seemed like a minute, and time was suspended.

When I went home that day I felt exhausted but unusually calm. I am not sure if I fully realized what had just happened. I was too tired. I knew, however, that I could finally rest, that there was no need to rush, no need to worry. The clock had stopped running.

SEVERAL DAYS LATER we were confident that the transplant was a success. The patient asked for a small handheld mirror, which she cautiously held up to her face. The corners of her mouth curved slightly upward and she gave her first smile with the transplanted face.

It was worth the long wait and it was worth all of the effort. The patient got a new life and a new face, and she was a silent hero of this historical moment.

You need a face to face the world.

APPENDIX

Face Transplant Surgery

The Cleveland Clinic was the first institution to approve facial tissue transplants from a donor to a patient whose face has been severely disfigured. While the dangers include life-threatening infections and the rejection of the transplant by the patient's immune system, the operation may be the only way to restore the function and semblance of a normal face.

Preparation Before Surgery

1. The candidate for the surgery is selected—e.g., a patient whose face was severely burned who is determined able to endure the surgery and a lifetime of anti-rejection drugs.

2. Blood vessels are clamped before surgery. Surgeons remove the patient's damaged skin. Muscles and nerves are retained.

Common Facial Damage

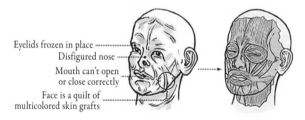

Eyelids frozen in place ·········
Disfigured nose ·········
Mouth can't open or close correctly
Face is a quilt of multicolored skin grafts

The Donated Facial Skin

1. Brain-dead donor of same sex and race is selected for donation. Recovered skin must be delivered within six to eight hours.

2. Facial skin is removed along with nerves and blood vessels. The flat and pliable tissue is called a flap.

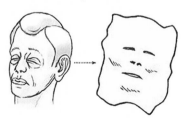

The Surgery

Surgeons position the donated skin, lining up openings for eyes, nose, and mouth. In an operation that may take 15 hours or longer, surgeons connect the blood vessels and nerves of the new tissue to those of the patient.

Microsurgery is performed under a microscope that provides magnification and illumination as surgeons reconnect the nerves and blood vessels.

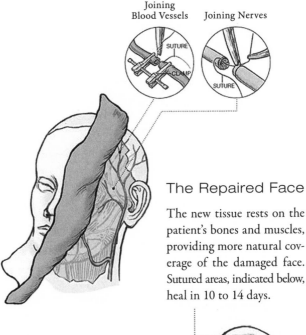

The Repaired Face

The new tissue rests on the patient's bones and muscles, providing more natural coverage of the damaged face. Sutured areas, indicated below, heal in 10 to 14 days.

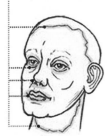

Source: Dr. Maria Siemionow, Cleveland Clinic

The diagram of the face-transplant sequence presented opposite and above was first published in the Science section of *The New York Times*, July 26, 2005.